The Consumer's Guide to

INVISALIGN®

Dustin S. Burleson, D.D.S.

Wasteland Press
www.wastelandpress.net
Shelbyville, KY USA

The Consumer's Guide to Invisalign
by Dustin S. Burleson, D.D.S.

First Printing – March 2013
ISBN: 978-1-60047-837-6

Printed in the U.S.A.

0   1   2   3   4   5   6   7   8   9   10

TABLE OF CONTENTS

INTRODUCTION

As an orthodontist, I see people every day who have questions about their teeth. They want to know what they can do to get the best possible smile. And after all, who can blame them? A beautiful smile is, well, beautiful! But there is a lot more to it than that - believe it or not.

Beautiful smiles come in all shapes and sizes, that is for sure. But the one thing that they usually all have in common is nicely aligned teeth. Even if others feel as though your smile is beautiful without having aligned teeth, you probably don't agree. And the person that you need to please is the one looking back at you in the mirror each day!

Many people seek information about how to get their teeth aligned properly, but most of those people want to avoid the old metal braces they saw kids wear during their youth. That's where Invisalign comes in handy.

Invisalign's technology offers a wide range of benefits to those who want the benefits of braces but without the neon sign pointing to their mouth to let everyone know that they are undergoing treatment.

That's where this book can help you. I wrote this book to give consumers a complete guide to Invisalign. Throughout the pages of this book, I aim to give you the ins and outs this revolutionary tooth-alignment system, how it works, and how to get started with it, should you choose to improve your smile.

My mission is to hopefully answer all your questions about Invisalign, and then some! After reading this book, you should be confident in your decision and comfortable with the treatment process.

Many people fear going to the dentist or orthodontist. Often times they aren't even sure why they have this fear. I believe it is because they don't always know what to expect once they get settled in the chair and the light moves in on them. I hope that this book helps to diminish those fears.

The more you know about the Invisalign system, including how it works, the more comfortable you will feel choosing it to improve your smile. I believe after you read this book you will agree with me that Invisalign is certainly a route worth considering!

CHAPTER ONE:
The History of Invisalign

If you are new to the idea behind Invisalign, you are not alone. While the concept of Invisalign is fairly new, the idea behind it has been a long time in the making. As you will soon learn, as technology has changed so too have the dental appliances being offered along the way.

One thing you are likely familiar with is the concept of aligning teeth. You may have even come across some people who have used the Invisalign method for aligning their teeth. But there's a good chance that when you think about fixing teeth to get them aligned, you picture metal braces.

Metal braces have been used in the dental industry for quite some time. There is no doubt that you can easily conjure up some images of people, usually school-aged, who don the shiny metal smile. While the metal braces did the job, and still do, many people find them to be a turn off and shy away from them.

Today, Invisalign allows people to use a virtually invisible route to straightening their teeth. This not only makes kids of all ages feel more confident and comfortable about the process, but it opens the door for millions of adults as well.

Yes, you read that right. Straightening ones teeth is not just for the adolescent, as many believe it is. There are many adults who have always wanted to correct their teeth but never got around to it, for whatever reason. The Invisalign System is a great way to achieve the results, without feeling like you have just taken a step back in time.

Adults that have always wanted to fix their teeth may not have wanted to walk around sporting some flashy metal braces. But Invisalign gives them the opportunity to straighten their teeth without everyone noticing or making a big deal out of it.

Plastic Dental Appliance History

The story of how Invisalign started begins with going back a few decades prior to the actual product, when thermoplastic sheets were emerging as a possibility in the world of dental appliances. If you have ever seen the plastic retainers that people wear, or used to wear, you will have an idea of how the plastic is used.

When thermoplastic sheets are heated to 250-450 degrees Fahrenheit, they will soften so that they can be formed.

Then, as the plastic cools, it retains the shape into which it was formed.

In 1959, a company by the name of The Tronomatic Machine Manufacturing Company of New York began making dental appliances with the thermoplastic sheets. The appliances they created were used in orthodontics, as well as in dental surgery, periodontics, restorative dentistry, and in some general dentistry practices.

Thus, an industry for plastic molded dental appliances was born!

An Idea is Conceived

Would you believe that an orthodontic patient invented Invisalign? It's true! A man by the name of Zia Chishti decided as an adult to undergo orthodontic treatment for crowding teeth. Using an overlay retainer, he was able to align his teeth. But he felt the process was slow and that there had to be a better way.

Chishti teamed up with fellow Stanford University graduate Kelsey Wirth and together they put their MBA degrees, and orthodontic knowledge, to use opening up a business known as Align Technology.

It was 1997, and they started the business in a Palo Alto, California garage. But don't let the foundation of starting in a garage fool you. Today, Align Technology's headquarters is in Santa Clara, Calif., and they have over 800 employees working in divisions throughout Costa Rica, Mexico, and Europe.

Come to think of it, there are several big corporations today that got their meager starts in a garage (e.g., Apple, Google, Mattel, Amazon, Microsoft, etc.). They must be on to something!

Technology Merged

What Chishti and Kelsey did was to essentially build upon the prior technology that was being used to make plastic dental appliances already. They took the idea, merged it with advanced ideas for alignment, and their concept was set into motion.

Invisalign uses the overlay concept for teeth alignment. But it adds in three dimensional technology. By using their concept, they created a system that will gradually move the teeth into proper positioning, one clear tray (aligner) at a time. Invisalign involves a variety of steps, which I will explain in more detail later in the book, including:

- Scanning the teeth.
- Making impressions of the teeth.

- Using a 3-D digital model of the teeth, using computer aided design (CAD) and computer aided manufacturing (CAM).
- Staging, where the treatment takes place.

The Invisalign System uses multiple appliances over a specific time period in order to achieve the desired results. The treatment plan created by the doctor will gradually move teeth to a specific area over time.

Each aligner is only worn for about two weeks, then it's time to move on to the next stage of the treatment plan with a new aligner. The aligners have all been designed to incrementally move the teeth into the desired position, a little bit at a time.

Through the use of technology, the Invisalign System has allowed people a host of benefits as a result. Who would have thought several of decades ago that there would one day be an invisible way to align teeth? Not many people would have been able to predict that one. But today, that's exactly what we have!

Getting to the Benefits

Little did the Invisalign founders realize that they would be creating a whole new ball game when it came to straightening teeth. Their creation has revolutionized the industry! It has given a new option to people that never wanted to consider metal braces. It has made straightening your teeth a discrete and more-comfortable process.

The best thing that has happened with the introduction of Invisalign is all the great benefits that it has provided. There has never been a better time to opt for teeth alignment than now. That's because the Invisalign System provides one of the most-convenient routes to teeth alignment that we have had thus far!

And since you are probably wondering, yes, the metal braces are still available. You may be wondering why, especially after you learn about all the advances in teeth alignment technology. The truth of the matter is that as an orthodontist I wish everyone would opt for the Invisalign route to alignment, but we just aren't there yet.

There are some people that still opt for the metal braces for a variety of reasons, it is what they are familiar with, it is cheaper, and they may not receive all the information they need about alternatives to metal braces.

Let's take a look at some of the benefits of using the Invisalign System, as opposed to going the route of the metal braces of yesterday.

First, let's look at some of the downsides of the metal braces:

- For starters, they are highly visible. This can make a lot of people feel uncomfortable and less than confident, especially in social situations.

- The metal braces are often a turn-off to those adults who are interested in aligning their teeth because they feel it would draw too much attention to the fact that they are undergoing treatment.

- Metal braces are often synonymous with being an adolescent, so like the point above, most people beyond adolescence find them to be undesirable.

- Metal braces need to be stabilized in order for the treatment to be effective. Problem is, there are times when the braces break loose from the teeth. This can give the teeth a chance to shift out of place. With Invisalign, there are no stabilization issues, so you are consistently on pace, working toward the treatment goals.

- Metal braces contain, well, a lot of metal. The problem with this is that the metal often irritates the mouth.

Broken wires, for example, can lead to a lot of discomfort and irritation.

- Metal braces do not get to come off the teeth during the treatment process. While there are adjustments made along the way, wearers of braces can't simply take them off for an hour and give their teeth a rest or a good flossing.

Beyond the metal braces, there is an option of ceramic ones. But they also come with their own cons that wearers often cite, including that they usually have to be worn longer, they are often larger than other braces, they can appear stained, they are more expensive than metal ones, and they are not as durable as the metal ones.

The good news is that the Invisalign System addresses all of these issues and more. The benefits of it are far reaching, including:

- Invisalign offers a discrete way to align the teeth. Patients no longer have to wear metal braces and wires that will send a signal to everyone that they undergoing treatment. This is especially beneficial to adults who have avoided fixing their teeth for years.

An invisible option allows patients of all ages to benefit from a beautiful set of straight teeth.

- Invisalign is a convenient way to align the teeth. One reason some people try to avoid having their teeth aligned is because they believe it is going to be disruptive to their lifestyle or inconvenient. But with Invisalign, people are able to live their life without the threat of disruption or being inconvenienced.

- Braces have typically always been associated with a certain amount of discomfort. Even with products available that aim to minimize that discomfort, people by and large find wearing braces on their teeth to be uncomfortable. Whether it is the metal poking into their mouth, the bands snapping off, or the ceramic being larger than they care for. Invisalign is a system that provides a more comfortable way for people to treat their teeth alignment issues. Patients report that their discomfort is minimal, if they have any at all. So Invisalign makes the entire experience more comfortable.

- Invisalign allows people to follow their normal hygiene routine. This is because, unlike other types of braces, the Invisalign appliance can be removed for about an hour per day. This is a huge benefit because it allows people to take a break if they feel they need it, as well as remove it to brush, floss, and even to enjoy the occasional sticky snack. With metal and ceramic braces, there are many foods that need to be avoided. That's not the case with Invisalign because you can remove them for the short time it takes you to eat.

- While the invisible nature that Invisalign provides is beneficial to those adults who want to align their teeth, it is equally beneficial to youths. No longer do they have to feel embarrassed or shy about showing up to school and flashing their smile. Even during the Invisalign treatment, those around them will likely not be aware they are wearing the appliance. This can help to prevent teasing and keep teens feeling confident.

- It is important to keep the mouth free of harmful plaque and bacteria. Traditional braces were problematic in this area, but Invisalign makes it easy for people to keep up on plaque removal. This simple benefit alone can help you avoid bad breath, tender or bleeding gums, mouth sores, and more. Invisalign can reduce your risk of infection around the gums, compared to braces, and is an important consideration for patients with heart disease or diabetes – as inflammation has been linked to these diseases.

- Invisalign treatment is incredibly accurate. The use of this 3D CAD/CAM technology has helped to create the desired results in less time.

- Poor brushing around metal braces can leave tooth discoloration, but people who opt for Invisalign do not have to worry about that issue. In fact, your doctor may be able to assist you with teeth bleaching either before, during, or after the Invisalign treatment process. Each doctor has their preference of when tooth whitening should be done, so be sure to inquire about the process.

- Invisalign also gives you the ability to see your treatment plan before beginning it. Through the use of advanced software, you can see what your teeth will look like. This will help ensure you get the desired results you are seeking and that your doctor recommends.

- Office visits for Invisalign alignment wearers is every eight to twelve weeks. Braces typically require more-frequent adjustments, so there is a greater possibility of less office visits with the Invisalign treatment process than with metal braces. Invisalign is an excellent solution for patients with a busy lifestyle.

- You will likely spend less time in the doctor's chair when you opt for Invisalign. There are no wires or brackets that need adjusting or fixing. Less time in the chair means more time to do all the other things you need to do. That's a good thing!

Benefits Beyond

As you can see, there are quite a few benefits to choosing the Invisalign System over metal and ceramic braces. But it is also important to discuss the benefits of having teeth aligned in the first place. Having properly aligned teeth can actually help you have better overall health, believe it or not. While most people don't see the connection between their oral health and their overall health, the two are linked together more than you probably realize.

When you have healthy gums and teeth, you are helping your body avoid infections, possible tooth loss, and periodontal disease. In fact, having an improper bite can be linked to difficulty chewing, headaches, and jaw problems. Crooked or crowded teeth can also make it more difficult to practice good oral hygiene and can lead to some of the serious health complications that have been mentioned.

The Future is Here

While Invisalign may have seemed like something that would be available in the future, the reality is that this exceptional product is here now. It's a convenient way to straighten and align teeth that simply involves snapping in clear aligners that have been custom fit to your mouth and treatment plan. About every two weeks a new aligner is used, helping to progress the treatment.

While we don't know exactly what the future holds in the field of orthodontics, I feel comfortable saying that the Invisalign System is a route that will help people achieve their desired alignment goals and do so in a nearly invisible manner. It's hard to beat that!

Let's Talk Cost

At this point you may be wondering about the cost of Invisalign. Fair enough. The average nationwide cost for Invisalign is around $5,000, so it is not much more than metal braces, and in some places it is right in line with them.

But that is just an average. The total cost really depends on your individual treatment needs. Some areas may offer it at around $5,000, while others charge as much as $10,000.

In some situations Invisalign can cost more than metal or ceramic braces. But that shouldn't be a reason to back away from it. Like most things in life, you get what you pay for, and high quality products and services tend to cost more.

Those who have opted to go with Invisalign have experienced first hand that the investment in the system is worth every penny. The benefits that people get from using the system far outweigh any concerns about it costing a little more.

Although the cost of Invisalign treatment varies with your treatment objectives and where you live in the country, the good news is that there are a variety of ways that you can get help paying for your treatment.

Some of the options to consider in paying for your Invisalign treatment include:

- **Payment plans.** Some doctors have arranged payment plan options, which will allow you to make monthly low interest payments to pay for the balance. Some payment plans offer no down payment options, as well as no interest. Inquire with your orthodontist to see what is offered.

- **Flexible spending accounts (FSA).** Many employers have FSAs options, where a designated portion of your paycheck would go into the account, allowing you to pay for Invisalign with pre-tax dollars. The funds are there to pay for qualified medical expenses. You can inquire to see if yours does, and if they do, if Invisalign treatment would be an option for getting payment assistance. A benefit of using a FSA is that the funds have not been subject to income tax, so it will save you a little bit of money in the long run.

- **Insurance assistance.** Check with your insurance provider. If they will not pay for the entire treatment, they may be willing to pay for a portion. Evening getting them to pay for a portion will be helpful. Then you can use one of the other options to fund the balance.

- **Other options.** If one of the above options are not ideal for your situation, you can always consider applying for health care financing through CareCredit® or other third party finance options, or you can save for it over the course of a year.

If you find after reading this book that you are interested in pursuing the Invisalign treatment route but feel finances are a concern, discuss your options with your orthodontist. Most orthodontists have information readily available to help you find a way to afford treatment.

The cost of Invisalign should not be a major issue, especially when you consider the exceptional and long-lasting treatment results that it provides. Metal braces may be slightly cheaper in most cases, but they come at a higher price that is paid to one's comfort, convenience, and confidence!

> *"I just started wearing my first set of trays this week. I'm so excited! I can't wait to see what the results will be after the Invisalign treatment is finished. This is so exciting!"*
>
> *– Richelle, Oregon*

CHAPTER TWO:
The Technology that Drives the Invisalign System

Bill Gates, of Microsoft fame, was once quoted as saying, "We're changing the world with technology." He may have been speaking about the products they were making, about computers, or about technology in general. Regardless, his statement couldn't be more accurate. He was right on, and even in the field of orthodontics, technology has changed everything!

The field of dentistry and orthodontics has grown tremendously thanks to technology. Today we have the ability to provide much more precise and thorough treatments and even be able to make adjustments along the away. When it comes to straightening teeth, Invisalign has taken the industry to a whole new level. Their use of technology has created a whole new segment of orthodontics. It's a segment that is able to provide advanced tooth alignment treatment and virtually guarantee incredible results.

Although, as pointed out in the first chapter, there were dental appliances being created out of thermal plastics, it wasn't until the creators of Invisalign came along that it was perfected and taken to the next level. Once they integrated the use of computer scanning and modeling into the equation, they ended up creating a system that has provided the best tooth alignment results thus far.

As a result, you and millions of other people have the ability to get the exact tooth alignment that you want and your doctor suggests you need. Once you see how the technology behind the Invisalign System has propelled the field of straightening teeth, you will probably be as impressed as I and many others in the field have been.

In the Beginning

When all of this advanced technology first got started, it wasn't nearly as advanced as it is today. The first patients to use Invalign also went through a process of laser scanning. But before the system was even made available to the public, the technology for this had advanced and a new scanning technique had been adopted. This new technique increased accuracy and precision.

The first step in the entire process of getting your teeth aligned is to have impressions of your mouth taken. In the beginning of the Invisalign method of alignment, the first impressions of a patient's teeth were done with polyvinyl siloxane (PVS), which at the time was the best route to providing accurate and stable impressions. Today there are PVS-based impressions and also digital scans that have made the process more efficient.

PVS-based impressions are still frequently used because they provide extreme accuracy, and the impression directly correlates to how well the Invisalign aligners fit the teeth. The impressions obtained provide the raw data that is used to create the aligners that you will wear to correct your teeth.

Once Align Technology, the creator of Invisalign, receives the PVS impressions or digital scan, they scan those impressions into a CT scanning machine.

Today's CT Method

The impression scanning method that is used today for Invisalign is referred to as "computerized tomography" or shortened to "CT" by most people. The nice thing is that the impressions of the teeth are scanned directly with the CT. This means that the process of pouring and encasing models of the teeth has been bypassed. Not only is it quicker to skip this process, but also the CT scan helps to make for a more accurate 3D model of your teeth.

With the CT providing such an accurate representation of the teeth, the information is stored in the computer. Along with the CT, your orthodontist will need to take what is called a "bite registration." This is important to show what your bite alignment is at the start of the treatment.

To get an idea of what a bite registration looks like, picture taking a big wad of gum, putting it in your mouth, and then biting down on it. When you take it out, or your doctor does, your bite registration will be found right in the gum. While we don't use a wad of gum to take your bite registration, thankfully, it does work as part of a highly accurate system overall.

Once Align Technology receives the impressions and bite registration their next steps are to create a "virtual" patient with that information. The impressions and information are all stored electronically, and the technician that is working on them will work with adjusting and digitizing the teeth. The clinician will follow this up by using a process that involves an "AutoBite" tool. All of this will help to create a perfect virtual model of the patient's mouth, which will be used to create the effective Invisalign treatment.

As you can see, there are several steps that are involved in leading up to the patient even getting the Invisalign aligners. Technology has made a lot of changes in process, but each of these changes has been in a direction that helps to make the system even more accurate. For example, the AutoBite tool entered the picture in 2003.

The development of this tool increased the bite set accuracy to 99 percent, and it also helped to reduce the lab setup time by some 80 percent. An increase in accuracy and a decrease in time is a win-win for everyone!

Consumers win when there is an increase in accuracy and effectiveness, as well as a decrease in time. Technology has seen some major changes in this area, all of which have lead to a more streamlined and precise alignment process.

The Staging Phase

While reading all this information on the process behind the Invisalign System may seem a little too technical for the consumer, it is important to at least have an overview of what goes on behind the scenes. By learning about each of these steps, you get an idea of just how much work goes into creating the Invisalign aligners.

People may sit in the orthodontist's chair for impressions and a bite registration, but behind the scenes, and before you start wearing your aligners, a lot of work has gone into creating them. And plus you just never know when this information could come in handy during a trivia game or conversation!

Once the technician at Align Technologies has put the impression and bite registration information into the computer system, a staging phase follows. During the staging phase, the technician will be creating the steps, or phase, in which the adjustments will be made to correct the teeth. Each of the phases that the technician creates will be helping to work toward guiding the teeth into the desired position.

Depending on the variation of treatment needed, this will help to determine the number of stages, or steps, that are required through the treatment process. The technician will also use the information gathered to help determine the timing of the movements of each tooth.

After the technician has completed the phasing stage, it is time to bring your doctor back into the picture. The staging, or treatment, file is then electronically forwarded to the clinician, where it will be reviewed before going forward. This review of the plan is referred to as a "ClinCheck."

Once the doctor has reviewed and approved the treatment plan, it is time for the aligners to be created, based on the specific treatment plan instructions. After the aligners have been created, the patient begins wearing them, getting a new aligner every two weeks as the treatment progresses.

The Invisalign Process

This graph provides a look at the steps that are involved in the Invisalign process, for the consumer, as well as Align Technology, where the aligner fabrication takes place.

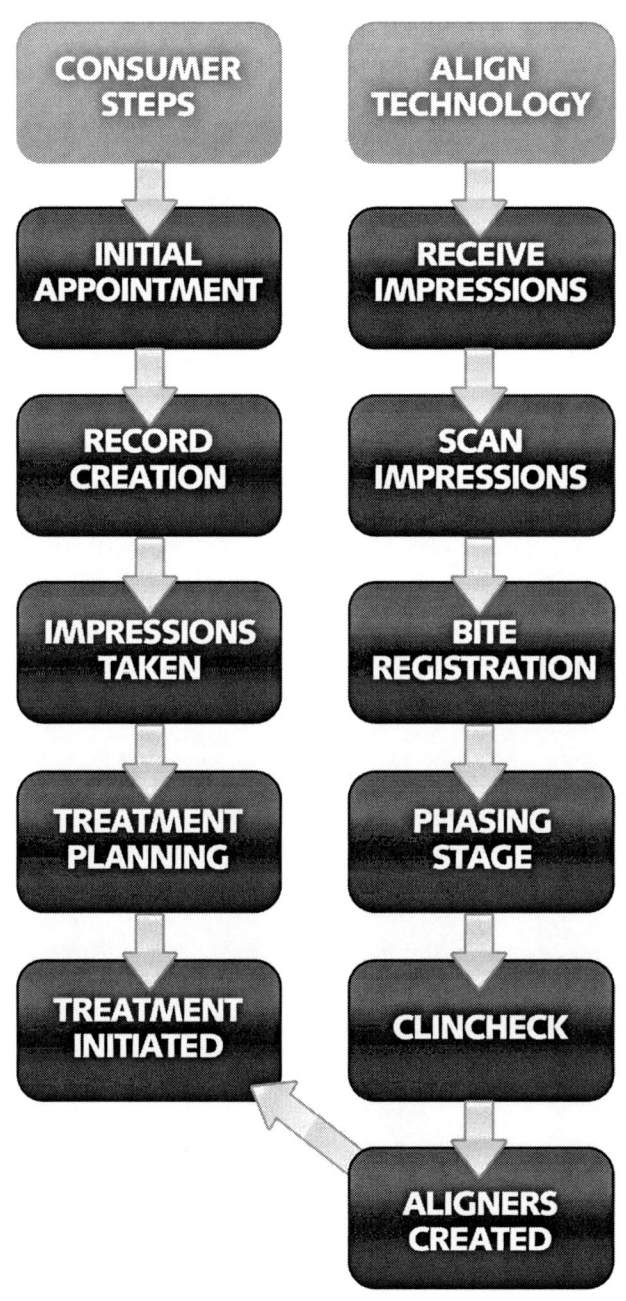

Consumer Confidence

In seeing just how much thought and work goes into the Invisalign process, it should bring consumers confidence that they are getting a treatment that is highly effective, as well as extremely accurate. The entire Invisalign process is quite in-depth, detailed, and impressive.

With all the technological advances that Align Technology has brought forward with the Invisalign System, it has brought a lot of benefits to the consumer. Let's take a look at some of the good things that have come out of all this for you, the consumer. While we have touched on some of these benefits previously, they are worth mentioning again because of the maximum comfort and effectiveness they provide.

- Aesthetics is one of the biggest benefits that consumers see when they evaluate Invisalign. That's because it provides an almost invisible route to straightening your teeth. Ceramic braces may also provide a look that is not as noticeable as the metal brace varieties, but there is a big advantage in that Invisalign is removable. So if you need to attend a party, take pictures, or you want to brush and floss normally, you can do so. Ceramic braces do not offer this convenience.

- With Invisalign being removable, it allows the patient to eat foods they would normally enjoy. They don't have to avoid any particular foods for fear that it will interfere with their braces.

- The advanced design of Invisalign has created a much more comfortable route to straightening the teeth. The plastic aligners are comfortable on the teeth and do not cause irritation, as some metal braces do to the cheeks and surrounding tissue. Patients also do not need to worry about wax or plastic sleeves, which are used with metal braces in order to help make it more comfortable.

- There is no need to worry about defects of the tooth caused by bonding to the enamel. Some people experience difficulty with getting metal braces to bond to their tooth enamel. Braces can also lead to tooth discoloration, which is also not an issue with Invisalign.

- The Invisalign system is effective in avoiding incidences of root absorption. With braces, root absorption can happen, it is believed because of the heavy force over the length of the treatment period. Root absorption is when the root of the tooth absorbs away. At this point there have been studies conducted by a couple of major universities in the country, and there have not been any incidence of root absorption when using Invisalign.

When there is root resorption present, the doctor must determine if it needs immediate treatment, such as a permanent bridge, or if the tooth is strong enough to withstand either for a short or long period of time. Invisalign, at least up to this point, has pretty much eliminated the threat of root absorption for those who want to have their teeth straightened.

- A unique benefit to using Invisalign is that the doctor has the ability to slow down the treatment, should it become uncomfortable. However, since patients typically report that they are comfortable with the Invisalign aligners, it hasn't been an issue. The Invisalign technology allows for such precision that if a patient does have a lower pain threshold, the treatment can be slowed down to compensate for it, making it more comfortable.

- Since Invisalign allows for normal routine brushing and flossing of the teeth, it helps to avoid gingivitis. Those who have braces usually find it more difficult to brush and floss, which can lead to higher risks of gingivitis, due to the poor oral hygiene. This is especially important for those adults who may have had experience with periodontal disease. Fixed appliances make it difficult to maintain good oral hygiene, something that Invisalign addresses because the aligner can be removed daily for brushing and flossing.

- For those that have large restorations and crowns, putting on fixed appliances, such as braces, can be problematic. There can be difficulty in getting the braces to bond to the teeth that have had crowns and restorations. To do so, the doctor usually has to use a porcelain primer and hydrofluoric acid, which can raise safety issues, as well as add a layer of unpredictability in the treatment process. With Invisalign, however, the technology allows for such a precise and unique treatment plan that even individual teeth, such as those with crowns or that have had restoration, can be aligned efficiently.

- Depending on the type of dental appliance that someone is using, their speech may be affected. For example, those who are using some types of retainers or quad-helix appliances will find that their tongue, or palate, is covered or irritated. This can lead to speech issues during treatment. The Invisalign aligners do not cover the palate or irritate the tongue, so there are no speech challenges.

- Invisalign saves a great deal of time for patients. For those who wear braces there is a lot of chair time because the braces need to be placed on the teeth, as well as the bands and wires. This can be a time-consuming process that keeps the patient in the chair quite a bit. The doctor also spends a lot of time working on adjusting the braces. When someone gets Invisalign, the chair time for the patient is significantly less because the aligners do not require numerous tools and parts to attach. For the doctor, Invisalign means less set-up time, as well as less time applying the aligners.

- The Invisalign aligners allow for vertical control, such as those who have a shallow overbite or anterior open bite. The aligners also reduce the risks of an open bite occurring during the initial leveling stages. The design of the aligners provides a bite block effect, providing excellent protection against open-bite and anterior open bite issues.

- Invisalign is also a system that requires less emergency appointments. With braces, if something goes wrong, the person is often in pain, such as being cut with a wire. This requires an immediate visit to the doctor. With Invisalign there are not usually emergency appointments because there is nothing that will cause such discomfort. If the person is in extreme discomfort, they can simply remove the aligner until meeting with the doctor.

- Even if a patient loses an aligner it is still not an emergency. Patients can wait until the next day to see the doctor for a lost aligner. With lost aligners, the patient may be advised to move on to the next one in the treatment phase, depending on where they are in the current phase when losing the aligner, or they may be told to wear their prior one. Another option would be that the doctor can get a replacement aligner within a couple of days time. So with Invisalign, unlike with braces, it reduces the risks for emergency office visits.

- A unique benefit to the Invisalign System is that the technology being used allows for specifying specifically which teeth are to be moved. Likewise, it allows for specifying which teeth should remain stable during the treatment process. This is especially important for those who have fixed partial dentures or teeth with preexisting root resorption.

- Invisalign offers another unique benefit, because it provides tooth protection from those who suffer from bruxism, or teeth grinding, whether at night or during the day. Because the aligner provides a protective barrier, it can prevent wear on the teeth that results from the grinding.

- For those who would like to bleach their teeth, Invisalign offers an ideal opportunity that will help them avoid the cost of having a plastic tray made specifically for bleaching. The bleaching can be done concurrently, using the Invisalign aligner. So once treatment has been completed, the patient will not only have straighter teeth, but they can be a lot whiter as well.

- Invisalign also offers benefits for specific people who may engage in sports or other activities. This is a feature that other tooth alignment appliances do not offer. For example, the person who plays a musical instrument (e.g., wind instruments, which require using the mouth) will be able to remove the aligner during the time they are playing, and the athlete can use the aligner as a mouth guard.

Invisalign uses stereolithography, or 3D layering, to create the aligners. Because we doctors have the ability to be a part of determining the treatment process, we can also show the patient the treatment plan as well. Patients have the ability to see the treatment plan at anytime before, during, and after the process. This is a benefit that helps the doctor, as well as the patient, feel confident about the plan, and it providing a successful outcome.

One of the advantages that Invisalign offers that I really appreciate as a doctor is the ability to redirect the course of movement mid-treatment, as well as to refine the treatment at the end. This helps ensure a successful outcome that braces and other such appliances simply cannot offer.

Invisalign is a 100 percent customized appliance that is different for every patient, providing a completely unique treatment plan for each and every person who uses the system. Because of this, it is just one more assurance that patients are getting an appliance that has been created especially for them to meet their individual needs.

As you can see, the Invisalign system offers a number of unique benefits that other dental appliances cannot provide when it comes to straightening the teeth. Technology has played a major role in advancing the entire process, making it more precise, as well as comfortable.

The Main Technological Advantage

There are many benefits that the Invisalign System offers. Perhaps the most significant one, however, is the technology itself. The technology allows for three-dimensional visualization. This allows the doctor to view the entire treatment plan, from beginning to end, before the treatment has even begun.

As a doctor, when I have the ability to view a patients entire treatment plan and see what the outcome will be, I feel confident knowing that my patients are getting the desired results. It's a system that provides precise results that are unmatched.

You simply can't get such accuracy and precision with other appliances and treatments for straightening the teeth. This makes it a significant advantage over other alignment treatment options.

> *"I have now completed an 18-month treatment of Invisalign trays. I'm happy with the results at this point. There are still a few small changes that need to be made, but those are barely noticeable. Two thumbs up for Invisalign!"*
>
> *– Vicky, Washington*

CHAPTER THREE:

How Your Doctor Works with the Invisalign System

When it comes to having straight teeth, there is a lot more that goes into it than patients usually realize. So far, you have gained a lot of insight into the in-depth process of how Invisalign works and the process that is used to create the aligners. Back in the doctor's office there is a lot that goes on as well. This is exactly what we are going to take a look at throughout this chapter.

Dentist or Orthodontist?

Many people who want straight teeth know that they need to go see a doctor. It's simply not something they can do at home. And let's face it, even if you could pull this off at home, it's probably not something you would want to try. Just thinking about that is enough to make you cringe. But we are fortunate to have many doctors in this country who are qualified to help you get the smile you deserve.

One of the common questions that people have when they go to seek tooth alignment treatment is whether they should see a dentist or an orthodontist. Most people are familiar with a dentist and what one does. But people are not quite as familiar with what an orthodontist does, and sometimes they may even have the wrong impression of them and what their focus is in their practice. That's what I aim to clear up here in discussing the difference between the two.

You may find that your dentist is prepared and offering to provide you with the Invisalign treatment. Many do offer it to their patients, but others still opt to go to the orthodontist for such a specialized treatment, and for good reason! Unlike a dentist, an orthodontist is a specialist at straightening teeth. An orthodontist has had 2-3 years of specialized education even beyond their years in dental school.

So when a dentist has graduated from dental school and is ready to get to work offering general dentistry to patients, those who wish to become an orthodontist continue on with their studies. They spend a couple of years intensively studying the process of straightening teeth; it's their specialty. When you choose to go to a dentist for Invisalign, you may be able to get the treatment itself, but you don't get that extra education and experience that comes with choosing an orthodontist.

An orthodontist has not only had the additional years of specialized education, but he or she has likely also worked with hundreds, if not thousands, of patients over the years. The experienced gained from working on straightening all of those patients' teeth is invaluable, and the patients reap the benefits.

The Doctor's Process

Now that you know why so many people opt for an orthodontist for their Invisalign treatment, it's a good time to take a look at just what we do once you contact us. This way you will have an idea of what we do in the doctor's office, in addition to what Align Technology does, which you learned about in the prior chapter.

There are some common steps in the Invisalign treatment process. We will take a look at each of these steps, so you have an idea of what happens and what you can expect out of each visit and step.

Step One

This first step is often when we meet the patient for the first time. Some may have already been a patient for other treatments, but many are new patients who are seeing us with the Invisalign treatment in mind. At this initial consultation, we determine if the patient is a good candidate for the Invisalign System. If the patient is a good candidate, we may go on to the second step at this time.

Most people are ready to move forward right then, while some may prefer to schedule the next step to take place at another appointment. Whether you are pressed for time or simply want to take a couple of days to think about it, your orthodontist and treatment coordinator will develop a plan that is just right for you.

Step Two

The next step is where we really get to know your teeth and gather the information that is needed in order for Align Technology to make the aligners for your treatment. To do this, we take photos and x-rays of your teeth, with impressions to follow. We already touched on the process of how impressions are taken in the prior chapter. It's kind of like taking a big wad of bubble gum or modeling clay and having you bite down on it, so we can get impression of what your teeth are currently like.

Taking these photos and impressions will provide Align Technology with the information they need to begin determining the best way to get your teeth straightened. While it may seem like a simple process, moving the teeth into proper position actually takes precise planning and involves important treatment decisions about every single tooth.

The x-rays that are taken are quite comprehensive. There is a series of x-rays taken so that we have images of every tooth and at all angles. We also take a panoramic x-ray of both the teeth and the mouth. This gives us the information we need about where the teeth are placed in the bone within the mouth.

The process of taking the x-rays runs around 15-20 minutes in all, but it is not something you want to rush. We need to be able to get good, accurate x-rays of all your teeth in order to ensure a successful treatment plan.

Once the x-rays have been taken, you will usually meet with the doctor so that an examination can be performed. At this time, we will also take digital photos of your teeth and mouth. These are taken at close range, as well as from a distance. All of this information gathered will be useful to the lab and in our office to help determine your treatment plan and progress.

We do the examination of your teeth prior to treatment because it is important to make sure you don't have any cavities or other issues that should be addressed prior to the Invisalign treatment. The more we know about your teeth, the better we are able to ensure a successful treatment outcome. Having all these photos also becomes a great resource for when the treatment has been completed. It will let you see the before and after progress from a variety of angles. Many patients love to see these photos once their treatment is complete, just so they can see the vast difference that the Invisalign System made.

The examination and process of taking the photos will probably take about another 20 minutes or so. This is also an ideal time for you to ask any questions you may have about the treatment process, assuming they haven't already been addressed prior to this appointment.

Step Three

For the next step you, the patient, are still in the office. No, we are not trying to keep you there as long as we can, even if it may seem like it. Trust us that while this all may take a little time out of your day it is a crucially important part of the treatment process. Your outcome will depend upon the accurate gathering of all this information.

Although your total appointment will probably run close to an hour and half, it is time well spent. The time is an investment in the future of your teeth. And plus, just think about all the time you are saving by choosing Invisalign over metal braces. You are still ahead when it comes to measuring the two, side by side.

In this next step we will get impressions of your teeth. To do this, we use a putty-like substance that is put into a tray. The tray is then put into our mouth, one for the upper teeth and one for the lower teeth. Once the tray is placed in your mouth, the putty-like substance forms around your teeth. It is a perfect copy of your teeth and bite. The impressions are an important component to the Invisalign System.

The impressions are sent to Align Technology, where they will use them to ultimately create the snug-fitting aligners that will be used to provide the corrective treatment to your teeth. The aligners are created so that you will change them every two weeks, wearing a new one that advances the treatment incrementally. The Invisalign aligners are created so precisely that you may not even realize that there is a difference in aligners, yet the teeth are still moving along, headed in the right direction the whole time.

Taking the impressions is a process that will also take about 20 minutes, but that time was already figured into the roughly 60 to 90 minutes you will spend getting everything in order. And trust me when I say that you will be having so much fun with all this that the time will fly by!

Step Four

Once we have the photos and impressions taken, we are ready to send them off to Align Technology, so they can use the information gathered in order to create the aligners that will be used for the treatment process. But before we do that, we have a computer system that we can use that will demonstrate for you what the treatment process will be like.

Through the computer program you will get a chance to see a digital image of what your treatment plan will look like, how it will progress through the stages, and what the final outcome will be. This is a great opportunity for both the patient and the doctor, and it's an advantage that some other forms of alignment treatments simply can't offer.

With the information gathered at your doctor's office, we can create that 3D image and give you a snapshot into the future. You can see what your teeth will look like during and after treatment. Not only will this make you feel eager to get started, but you will know where your journey leads before you even take the first step.

Step Five

You are already familiar with what happens once all of your information reaches the Align Technology lab, since it was discussed in the prior chapter. It usually takes 1-2 weeks for them to create your aligners, based on the information provided. Once the aligners are created, you will come back for an appointment where you will get your first aligner, as part of your Invisalign starter kit.

In your starter kit, you will find your first upper and lower aligner. What comes inside your Invisalign starter kit will vary by orthodontist, but it will contain your new aligner, cases to store them in, and most likely a brochure about getting started and caring for your aligner. Some starter kits may also come with such items as a new toothbrush, floss, a special cleaning brush, toothpaste, and possibly even some cleaning samples.

In your Invisalign Starter Kit, there will be two cases, one red and one blue. You have two different colors so that you will be able to tell the current and previous aligners apart. Whenever you remove your aligners, whether for cleaning your teeth or to take a break for some other special reason, you will store them in the color-coded cases.

Once you get your starter kit, this is where the excitement begins, as your tooth alignment journey really gets down to business. The prep work has been done, and you are ready to start wearing the aligners and progressing through the stages that have been created for your treatment.

The Typical Process

While this process is what many orthodontists follow, it is important to realize that not everyone works exactly the same way. Some doctors may do things a bit differently or in a different order, but in the end, we all aim for the same result, which is to help our patients achieve straighter teeth.

Typically speaking, however, most orthodontists will follow a basic three-step procedure to get patients started in the process. There are more steps that don't involve the doctor, but there are three common ones that involve the patients in order to get started with their Invisalign treatment.

These first three appointments that you can expect include:

1.   Initial consultation or exam.

This is the initial exam to see if you are a good candidate for the Invisalign treatment system. This is an ideal time to bring along a list of any questions you may have. Don't be afraid to take the time you need to get all of them answered. We want you to feel comfortable with the treatment and know exactly what to expect. Ideally you would have read this book, since it can obviously provide a lot more information that a doctor can in one office visit. But either way, be sure to ask lots of questions so you understand everything from the cost of the procedure to what type of outcome you can expect.

2.   Exam and Information Collecting.

During the second visit, you will have your exam with the doctor, along with the x-rays, photos, and impressions that will be taken of your teeth and mouth. The order that this will take place depends on the doctor you are visiting. But all this will be accomplished at the visit, regardless of the order in which it is done.

3. **Aligner Time.**

At the third appointment with the doctor, you will receive your first set of aligners. You will leave there with your aligners and information on what to do with them, how to clean them, etc. This is the time you will get your Invisalign Starter Kit and your teeth will begin to start making its progress toward a successful transformation and new smile.

Individual Additions

As the Invisalign treatment process begins, most people fit into the above mentioned steps without any other issues. However, sometimes there are people who need additional steps before being able to wear their aligners. Those steps may involve the doctor needing to have small spaces created in between the teeth. This process is called interpoximal reduction.

The reason that some patients need to go through the interpoximal reduction step is that their teeth are extremely crowded. If extreme crowding is an issue, then your doctor will discuss this process with you. It usually takes under an hour to create the necessary spaces. The process is not painful. It's a normal step for those with extremely crowded teeth and involves removing a small amount of the outer tooth enamel in order to provide more space between the teeth for proper alignment.

The interpoximal reduction process is also sometimes referred to as reproximation, enamel reduction, stripping, or slenderizing. If your doctor feels you need this done due to the overcrowding, he or she will explain the procedure and answer all your questions regarding it. This is simply one more step that is used for some patients to help ensure a successful treatment outcome.

Additionally, as mentioned before, there may be some people who need to have cavities filled prior to Invisalign treatment, and some people may need to have tiny attachments bonded to a tooth here and there, if the tooth needs to be rotated. These are all issues that your orthodontist will address with you in an effort to provide you with the best possible treatment, as well as outcome.

Behind the Scenes

While the above steps give you an idea of how the doctor is involved in getting your Invisalign treatment process started, it doesn't give you the whole story. Behind the scenes there are many people working to help design, create, and eventually bring your aligners to the orthodontists' office.

The software program that is used to help make the Invisalign treatment process so successful is called ClinCheck. The ClinCheck software allows for the input of all the initial information that the doctor has collected, and it is used to create the 3D virtual file. The file is a representation of what the doctor's treatment plan is going to be for that patient.

Once Align Technology gets the information we provide and they put it into their database and create a treatment plan that will give us the desired results, the doctor is involved again. Only the patient doesn't need to be present for the next step.

This is a step that just involves the doctor, whereby Align Technology will provide the doctor with the computer imaging treatment plan, or ClinCheck, for each patient. In order for the ClinCheck report to be provided to the doctor, there is first a "staging" process that the technician works through. The technician first scans in all the images and impressions that were provided by the doctor. Then they are used to "stage" or virtually place the teeth in their final position. For this to be accurate, it is essential that all the reporting, x-rays, images, and impressions sent from the doctor be accurate.

The ClinCheck review gives the doctor the chance to review the treatment plan and make sure that he or she agrees with every aspect of it, including that which has been designed in the treatment software. The treatment program is used to help create the ClinCheck files.

The treatment program is used to virtually position the teeth and work through the staging process of the treatment plan. This software is just one step in the advanced technology that is used to create the Invisalign aligners. The technician who uses the software has been trained not only in how to use it, but also in orthodontic practices and principles.

Using the software and information, the technician creates a "Treat file," which is then turned into the ClinCheck file that the doctor will review prior to the aligners being fabricated.

The Staging process is where the actual plan for moving the teeth takes place. Each tooth is looked at individually and a plan is created for getting it perfectly aligned. They start with a reference number of "0" for each tooth, with the goal of getting it to a "1" when treatment is completed. When it reaches the "1" reference number, then it has successfully completed treatment.

Having these reference numbers helps the technician move forward with using a staging editor software to calculate the ideal tooth movement distances and the amount of overlap between teeth through the entire sequence. This advanced technology helps to ensure that your teeth will be moved at an ideal pace in order to maximize the success of the overall outcome.

When the doctor receives the computer treatment plan for each of his or her patients, they will need to review it to ensure it meets the goals they have discussed with and planned with their patient. Only after the doctor has given the approval of the treatment plan will Align Technology go forward to the next step of creating the custom aligners.

Beginning the Treatment

Once all the prep work has been completed and the aligners have been fabricated, the patient is ready to begin the actual treatment phase. Throughout the entire treatment, the doctor will want to schedule an appointment to see the patient every 8-12 weeks. This is to make sure that the treatment is progressing as it should and that there are no issues.

These scheduled appointments will continue throughout the duration of the treatment plan. The length of time that the treatment will take varies by person, but it is about 9-12 months for the average adult. This is a significant advantage over metal braces, which usually require 18-24 months to complete treatment.

Invisalign, as noted before, is a much quicker route to completing tooth alignment treatment. It will also usually require spending quite a bit less time in the doctor's chair for check-ups and maintenance.

Trusting the Process

As you can see, there is a lot that goes into the Invisalign treatment process, both behind the scenes and alongside the patient. The good news is that this is a system that has been perfected over time. In fact, to date there have been well over 1.5 million people who have used the Invisalign System with exceptional results.

With so many people having used Invisalign, it should bring people comfort in knowing that all the "bugs" have been worked out. When there are new things being used in any field there are sometimes issues that need to be worked out before everything is perfected. The number of people are in the millions, each of whom are getting a series of anywhere from 20-40 total aligners throughout the course of their treatment.

With Invisalign, so many people have used it that the system of gathering information, creating aligners, and providing excellent results has been perfected and usually runs like a well oiled machine!

"I'm so excited! I have just seven more weeks left of aligners and then we begin the refinement process. I'm so happy with the way the results are shaping up!"
– Marylee, California

CHAPTER FOUR:
How the Invisalign System Works for You

As you can see thus far, the Invisalign System offers many advantages over other tooth alignment options. For those that have already chosen to go the Invisalign route, they know, feel, and see the difference it has made in their lives. For the person who wants to have a straighter, more beautiful smile, it is hard to beat what Invisalign has to offer and what it can do for you.

What Invisalign Offers You

While you have spent some time reading and learning about how the Invisalign System was created and how it works to straighten your teeth, you are likely most interested in what advantages it can offer you personally. Most people want to know how the system will work for them, so they can ensure that it is the right route to take for their treatment.

After all, it is what it will do for you that will help you feel comfortable about your decision to go with Invisalign, if you choose to do so. Knowing how it was created and the technology behind it is helpful and interesting, but from a consumer's perspective, it's more important that it is esthetically pleasing, for example.

In this chapter, we are going to look at all of the benefits that you, the consumer, will gain from choosing the Invisalign System, as opposed to other alignment options. We will take a look at all the things it does to work for you!

Looking Good

Aesthetics is likely one of the biggest reasons that consumers choose to go with Invisalign. The sheer fact that you won't have to walk around for a year or two wearing traditional metal braces is a huge benefit. With Invisalign, most people will have no idea that you are undergoing treatment because it has been designed to be invisible.

You can wear your Invisalign aligners throughout your treatment without drawing attention to the fact that you are straightening your teeth. While this is a great benefit for those teens who may still be in school because it can help them avoid being teased and help make them feel more confident, it's also great for adults.

Prior to the introduction and popularity of Invisalign, millions of adults wanted and had considered tooth alignment, but refused. They simply didn't want to wear traditional metal braces. Now that the Invisalign System is available, there are many adults who choose to straighten their teeth on a regular basis. No longer do people have to wish that they had gotten their teeth straightened as a teen because Invisalign is available to a wide range of people, regardless of age.

With the Invisalign System, you can feel confident, comfortable, and not have to worry about what others may think or draw unnecessary attention to yourself. Invisalign allows you to continue your normal routine, including going to work and interacting with friends and family, all while conveniently and discretely straightening your teeth.

The esthetic appeal of Invisalign alone is one that is difficult to beat, simply because it is such a great benefit to consumers, regardless of age. When it comes to the aesthetics, you have to really ask yourself if you would rather walk into work, school, or other places and flash a smile that looks like your teeth or one that has metal braces. Most adults, at least, can't imagine the latter, and most teens would agree as well.

Comfort Counts

One of the concerns that many orthodontic patients have is whether or not it will be comfortable. This is a legitimate concern, and it is important to discuss this, no matter what route you take for treatment. You need to know what to expect and get some honest information about what the discomfort level will be.

When it comes to metal braces, as we've touched on already, there is a higher potential for discomfort. There always has been. People have been searching for ways to try to make them less painful for quite some time now. But the truth of the matter and bottom line is that you are putting metal wires into your mouth. This in and of itself is bound to create some discomfort.

Metal braces create a lot of discomfort for people because the metal wires can end up poking into the sides of the mouth. People can have broken or loose wires, which may lead to an orthodontic emergency. There are also issues that arise with loose bands, which can result from eating hard or sticky foods, or even from playing with the braces. From wires that poke and cause soreness, to a sore and achy mouth and teeth, most patients experience some level of discomfort with metal braces.

Another issue with metal braces is that many people complain of a pressure that they feel once the braces are on their teeth. This may prompt them to keep touching and playing with the braces, which could lead to further problems, such as the bands coming loose.

Even those who choose to go with ceramic braces find that there is a certain level of discomfort that comes along with them. Many people complain of pain. They can also be more difficult to remove, causing additional discomfort, and they are more susceptible to breaking easily, which means more visits to the orthodontist for repairs.

With the Invisalign System there is some discomfort, as there is with all types of tooth alignment treatment, but most patients report that it is minimal. During the first week patients usually find that they experience the most discomfort with their aligners. This is because it is new, and they are just getting used to having the aligner on their teeth. After about a week, however, patients find that they are used to them and the discomfort is very minimal, if they have any at all.

Each time you get a new aligner, you may find that your teeth feel a little sensitive for the first 24 hours. This minimal amount of discomfort is normal and usually subsides once you get used to the new aligner. Plan on 1 or 2 days of discomfort. With Invisalign, you also have the ability to remove the aligners for an hour or so each day, so if you are finding that there is any discomfort on these particular days, you can always take a break by removing them for a short period.

Another important aspect to comfort when it comes to Invisalign is that it is not made of metal. It is made from a smooth plastic that will not have sharp edges or cut into the mouth. Those who use the system typically do not have issues with the way the aligners feel in the mouth, as they have been designed to maximize comfort for the wearer.

It would be great if we lived in a world where we could move your teeth and you wouldn't feel a thing throughout the entire process. But that's simply not the case. Your teeth are actually being moved into the desired position, so a slight discomfort is to be expected. The majority of people who use Invisalign find them to be comfortable enough that they remain satisfied with their decision throughout the treatment process.

Even if you find there is a slight discomfort with using Invisalign, it is still the most comfortable option for tooth alignment available today. From less time causing pain in the mouth, to less pain of having to sit in the orthodontist's chair, it is the most comfortable option on the market. And the results will be long lasting and completely worth your time and effort.

Hygiene Helper

You may be aware that it is important to brush and floss your teeth daily, but you may not be aware of all the problems that can result if you don't. The truth of the matter is that your oral hygiene can actually have an impact on your overall health. Your oral health even has an impact on your heart health, believe it or not!

Gingivitis is a common condition that can result from poor dental hygiene. Crowded or misaligned teeth may be more difficult to clean, especially in between them, which will allow the plaque to build up.

Periodontal disease involves inflammation and infection that can wreak havoc on your teeth, gums, tooth sockets, and even periodontal ligaments. The symptoms include swollen and tender gums, a sore mouth, and bright red or bleeding gums. In other words, getting gingivitis can lead to a lot of problems with your teeth. But it has an impact on more than just your teeth.

Researchers have found that there is an association between gingivitis and heart disease and that the vast majority of people who have cardiovascular disease also have some form of periodontal disease.

The correlation on heart disease and gingivitis is still being researched so they can determine exactly what the connection between the two is. However, with all that we know about what can result from improper brushing and flossing, it makes it that much more important to not only make the commitment to get your teeth aligned so that you can properly brush and floss and remove plaque between teeth, but to continue properly cleaning your teeth during treatment.

The only tooth alignment system that allows you to continue properly brushing and flossing your teeth each day is the Invisalign System. The Invisalign System takes the issue of proper cleaning out of the equation. Braces, whether metal or ceramic, make it difficult to continue brushing and flossing properly during treatment. They make it difficult brush, floss, and remove the plaque between the teeth. Braces also increase the chances that food can become trapped in between the teeth because the braces and wires act as a barrier, trapping food and bacteria.

With the Invisalign aligners, you can remove the aligner each and every time you need to clean your teeth. So there are no issues with proper cleaning. You can go about your normal brushing and flossing routine by simply removing your aligners. And if you don't have a normal routine of brushing and flossing, then now is the perfect time to get started. When the aligners are gone and your brand new beautiful smile is finished, your teeth are clean and well taken care of.

Your tooth alignment is an investment in yourself and you want to make sure you brush and floss properly in order to help protect that investment!

Convenient for Your Schedule

We live in busy times today, and if there is one thing that people want, it is convenience. This is evident by all of the fast food restaurants on every corner in just about every town, as well as in all the pre-packaged foods that are lining the store shelves across Any town U.S.A. We all want convenience because let's face it –we have a lot of things we need to do, and we don't always have a lot of time to get them done.

While it may not be ideal to hit the fast food restaurants or buy pre-made processed foods in an effort to save time, there are some legitimate ways we can save time in our lives. When it comes to straightening your teeth, there are decisions that can make you spend more time in the doctor's chair and be a lot less convenient for you, and there are choices that will help eliminate some of these additional visits and will be much more convenient for you in the long run.

Metal braces, for example, have traditionally been a route that required frequent doctor visits. And those are just the ones that are scheduled. There are also additional emergency visits in order to deal with the broken and loose wires, or other issues that can arise.

Metal braces, as well as ceramic ones, will usually require more office appointments and more time in the chair for repairs and routine treatment maintenance. They are not exactly what you would call convenient. Ask anyone who has had metal braces how often they visit the doctor, for both planned and unplanned visits, and see how inconvenient it was for them to take off of school or work to stop in for brace issues.

With the Invisalign System, you will have some doctor's visits. That's to be expected because after all, you are undergoing treatment. That alone requires you to see a doctor to ensure that your treatment is progressing as planned or if any adjustments need to be made. But what you will find with

Invisalign is that it is a much more convenient system all the way around.

Invisalign will not require a bunch of emergency visits. There are no brackets and wires to come loose or break. You will have your normal visits in order to pick up a new aligner. If you needed to see the doctor in between then for something, you can make an appointment, but it is not likely that you will have many additional appointments like these. Emergencies are not an issue with Invisalign.

Also, the length of time you wear Invisalign is typically much less than with other forms of tooth alignment. So while you may be going to routine appointments for a year or less with Invisalign, you would likely be wearing metal or ceramic braces for a couple of years. That's a lot more time devoted to appointments with braces, as compared to Invisalign.

The most ideal option for tooth alignment for those who are seeking convenience is the Invisalign System. It's convenient in terms of how long you will be in the doctor's office, but it's also convenient in that you can remove them if you need to for short periods of time. It is a system that provides advanced treatment, delivers remarkable results, yet gives people the convenience they so badly need in their lives.

Getting Social

Whether you are someone who likes to chat it up with everyone around you or you prefer to sit alone with a book, you will no doubt want to feel confident in whatever you do. Confidence is a major key component to leading a successful life. It was Henry Ford who was quoted as saying, "Whether you think you can or think you can't, you're right." This is so important because it is how we see ourselves and believe in ourselves that helps lead us down the path to success.

In all areas of your life where you have a choice, you will want to make choices that lead you down the path of having the most confidence. The more confident you feel, the better you will likely perform in just about any area of your life. Believe it or not, this even pertains to straightening your teeth!

Many people who do not have straight teeth tend to be less confident. They don't like to smile or may even cover their mouth when they smile. They take pictures and keep their mouth closed. They try to avoid having anything to do with showing their teeth to people, all because they are lacking confidence. Not having a beautiful smile that gives you confidence can be a real problem in your life.

There are a lot of people that simply choose to have their teeth aligned because of confidence. They want to like what they see when they smile, or feel good about showing others their smile or teeth when they are speaking. Nothing wrong with that, but as an aside, they still gain all the health benefits of having aligned teeth as well. This is a major theme of my book "Stop Hiding Your Smile! A Parent's Guide to Confidently Choosing an Orthodontist."

Now that you know how important a confident smile is to just about everyone on the planet, think about what would make someone feel more confident. Would it be someone who walks into a room and smiles to show a full mouth of metal braces, or someone who smiles and nobody can even tell that they are wearing Invisalign aligners to straighten their teeth?

Even if your teeth have not reached the desired position yet, you will feel more confident in the Invisalign aligners, simply because the other ones are drawing more attention to the person's mouth, and they didn't feel confident about it to begin with.

People tend to feel much more confident when they can undergo tooth alignment using the Invisalign System. Rather than feeling embarrassed and not wanting to smile, they can feel confident and not mind smiling and talking. Besides, each week their treatment is getting closer to completion, and their teeth are getting straighter. So they will increasingly be feeling more confident as the treatment progresses.

This is important for just about every age group that is considering tooth alignment. Teens who have been advised that they should have tooth alignment will feel better about going to school and continuing their normal activities wearing Invisalign.

While it's not a pleasant thing, the reality is that we live in a society where there is a lot of teasing that goes on. It's not a new concept, as there has always been some teasing that took place in schools, even when I was growing up. But today, kids seem to be merciless in their teasing.

If you can help your child avoid this by choosing Invisalign, you will be helping them build confidence and avoid some social issues that can be uncomfortable. The same goes for adults. Most adults who want to straighten their teeth would usually shy away from it because they didn't want to have the metal braces or for people to know they were undergoing treatment. Invisalign allows adults to continue with their normal jobs and lives, without having to feel embarrassed about the fact that they are straightening their teeth.

All the way around, the Invisalign System is a great tool for helping people feel more confident during their tooth alignment treatment process. And feeling more confident is always a good thing!

Seeing is Believing

Another great way that Invisalign works for you is to show you the final anticipated results ahead of time, before you start treatment. When you choose to have braces, you are not likely to get such insight into how well your teeth will turn out once treatment is over. But with Invisalign, the technology has made it such a precise treatment that it is possible for us to show you what your teeth will look like once the plan for alignment has been followed.

Being able to see the process, as well as the final outcome, is a great way to feel confident about making the Invisalign decision. Rather than not knowing what you will get and what the results will be, your doctor can give you a good look at what your smile will be like once you finish treatment. Seeing really is believing, and it's just one more way that the Invisalign System works for you!

Discussing and Considering Invisalign

As you read through the pages of this book, you are learning a great deal about not only Invisalign, but about other alignment options as well. It may be helpful to answer a few questions about your own experience and goals in order to help make the determination of whether or not you would like to choose Invisalign.

Give these questions some thought when making your decision about which type of application is the best route for your treatment. If you are parent who is reading this book and considering Invisalign for your teenager, consider these questions from the point of view of your teen, or discuss them with your son or daughter.

They are the ones that will be going through the treatment, so it is good to have an open conversation about how they will feel with each treatment option you are considering.

1. How important is aesthetics to you throughout your treatment? Could you better see yourself wearing metal braces in social settings, or would you rather have a treatment option that is more invisible?

2. How concerned are you with comfort when it comes to your tooth alignment treatment? Does the thought of having metal brackets and wires poking into your mouth worry you? Do you prefer to be able to have the option to take the appliance off for an hour or so each day in order to get a break from it all together?

3. How concerned are you about oral hygiene? If you are wearing metal braces, for example, does it concern you that you may have difficulty properly brushing and flossing your teeth for a couple of years? Would you rather have a treatment appliance that can be removed each day in order to provide proper oral hygiene?

4. How concerned are you about having the ability to continue eating whatever you would like? Are you

concerned that with metal braces you may have to give up eating things that are sticky, gummy, or that may interfere with the wires and brackets? Or would you rather have a system like Invisalign, which allows you the ability to temporarily remove the device in order to eat a snack or meal?

5. How concerned are you about social confidence when it comes to the process of straightening your teeth? Would you feel confident going about your normal daily activities with metal or ceramic braces that people can see? Or would you rather have a tooth straightening device, such as Invisalign, that provides a nearly invisible treatment option?

6. How concerned are you about convenience when it comes to teeth straightening treatment? Are you okay with having to go for many appointments over the course of a couple of years, including some emergency office visits due to broken brackets and wires, like with metal braces? Or would you rather not only shorten the time that the entire treatment process takes, but also cut down on the number of office visits all together, such as with Invisalign?

7. How concerned are you with having the ability to see what your teeth will look like once treatment is

complete? Are you more comfortable going with a treatment option, such as Invisalign, where you will not only have the ability to see what your teeth will look like once the treatment has been completed, but also uses advanced technology to offer a more precise and customizable treatment plan all together?

Take some time to consider the questions above. They are a great way to really get yourself thinking about what option is best for you. And again, if you are a parent who is considering Invisalign for your teenager, think about the questions and discuss them with him or her. Discussing these questions together will give you some great insight as to what type of treatment plan really is the best route for you and your family.

"After evaluating both braces and Invsalign, I decided to go with Invisalign. There are so many more benefits to the system, and it's so much more advanced. I feel confident that the process will be smooth and the outcome will be great!"

–Roxanne, Florida

CHAPTER FIVE:
Popular Questions About Invisalign

As an orthodontist, I get plenty of questions about Invisalign. Everyone has questions ranging from the cost to how long it will take and everything in between. And there's nothing wrong with that. Not at all!

I'd rather people feel completely comfortable with their decision, and the only way to do that is to ensure that all their questions have been answered. The more you know and understand the entire Invisalign process, the more comfortable you will feel making it your preferred treatment choice.

This chapter is going to focus on answering some of the most popular questions that I get about Invisalign. While I can't list every question that I've been asked, simply because it would take a lot of space and I may not be able to remember each one, I am going to focus on the most popular ones. If quite a few others have this question, there is a good chance you may as well. Hopefully, this section will help answer many of those questions you have about Invisalign.

Q. Does Invisalign really work?

A. Many people want to know if Invisalign really works. I think this is a question that arises because the system is virtually invisible. They have this idea in their head that if they can't "see" it doing something on the teeth, then perhaps it is not really working. With metal braces, for example, people can "see" that something is happening. Perhaps they don't really know if is working and really aligning the teeth, but because the braces are so visible, they assume it must be working. Rest assured that with Invisalign the treatment is absolutely working.

The fact that it is an invisible treatment is an aesthetic perk. It allows you to have treatment without making a statement about it all the time. Plus, the Invisalign system uses the most advanced technology in order to align your teeth. It is a precise and completely customizable treatment route that gives excellent results.

Q. How many people have had Invisalign?

A. At the time of writing this book, there have been over 1.5 million people who have used the Invisalign System to align their teeth. This number increases exponentially each year. As people increasingly hear about all the benefits of the treatment option, they often choose it. It has quickly become one of the most popular dental appliances in the world.

Q. Would veneers make an ideal alternative to Invisalign?

A. Some patients wonder if veneers would make an ideal alternative to getting Invisalign. Veneers are the equivalent to putting a bandage over a sore. They may cover up the problem, but they don't actually address the root of the issue. With veneers, you simply put a facing or covering over what you don't want people to see, but the problem is still there underneath.

Another issue with veneers as an alternative to Invisalign is that they need to be replaced. Some people find they need to replace their veneers every 6 to 12 years. So with veneers, there is going to be ongoing pain, discomfort, and costs each time this work needs to be re-done. Invisalign is a noninvasive alternative that does <u>not</u> involve cutting on tooth structure.

Q. How much does Invisalign cost?

One of the first things that people want to know is how much the Invisalign treatment will cost them, and how much it will cost versus getting metal braces. This is a legitimate question, there is no doubt. You should always know what the cost of any procedure is going to be, so you can account for that and know what to expect.

With Invisalign, it really matters where you are seeking it geographically. Typically speaking, the cost for Invisalign treatment ranges from $5,000 to $10,000. On average, the cost is right around $6,000. But some areas of the country may cost more, while others cost less.

This difference in cost is largely impacted by and reflective of the cost of living in the different geographic areas. For example, you could probably expect to pay more for Invisalign if you are getting it in New York City than if you are getting it in Akron, Ohio. That's because the doctor is going to have a lot higher expenses being in New York City than one does being in Akron, Ohio. But on the flip side, the average salaries in areas are also in line with what is being charged, in that those in New York City are likely making more on average than those living and working in Akron.

No matter where you live and what the cost, consider the lifelong returns of a great smile and healthy bite. For a life-changing smile, I personally know many adults who have told me they would have spent multiples of the treatment cost, had they known what a difference a new smile would make in their lives!

Q. Does my insurance cover Invisalign treatment?

A. This is a question where the answer really lies with your insurance company and what they provide. Each insurance provider is different, so the best way to find out the answer to this question is to contact your insurance provider and ask them about your policy. I have found that while insurance companies don't typically pay for the whole treatment, they do often cover a portion of the total expense.

Even if you end up getting a portion of it covered by insurance, it is better than nothing, and it also helps to lower the total cost that you would be spending on metal or ceramic braces. Some insurance companies offer $500-$1,500 toward the Invisalign treatment. Contact yours to see what they are willing to contribute toward your treatment.

Q. What are my payment options if it's not covered by insurance?

A. Determining what route you will take to pay for your Invisalign treatment is a common concern for many patients. But there are options, so the best thing to do is make a list of all the possibilities and then explore each one of them. First, you will want to check with your orthodontist to see what financial options are offered. Many orthodontists offer payment plans to help you with your treatment.

Additional routes to paying for your Invisalign treatment include flex spending accounts, third party financing, or saving up for a year and then initiating the treatment. By being creative, most people do find a route to paying for Invisalign with which they are comfortable. It's just a matter of exploring your options and deciding which is the best route for you.

Q. *How does the cost of Invisalign compare with the cost of metal braces?*

This also depends on where you live. Location helps determine even what you will pay for metal braces. When comparing the price of metal braces with the price of Invisalign, it's important to compare like-markets. Your best option is to check with your orthodontist to see what he or she charges for both.

I would recommend comparing the options beyond just the total cost. Most people find that the benefits of Invisalign are worth the little extra that it costs to have it as their preferred treatment route.

Along with comparing the benefits, it is important to also note that if you spend more time visiting the orthodontist due to having metal braces, you will incur more expenses. Even having to drive back and forth, and possibly take additional time off of school or work, all add to the overall treatment expense.

It's important to keep these additional expenses in mind because when you get a quote for the various types of treatment options, you will just hear bottom line figures, rather than what all goes into that figure or may add to it at some point. It's important to weigh more than just the overall cost because there is a lot more involved than just the initial cost.

It is important to also take into account the benefits when considering the costs. As you have learned through the prior chapters, the Invisalign System uses advanced technology that has made the tooth alignment process precise and customizable. These benefits alone are worth any additional costs. After all, getting your teeth aligned is an investment in yourself.

You want to make sure that if you are going to invest money into straightening your teeth, no matter how much it is, that you get the best possible results and are satisfied with the outcome. Those who get Invisalign are pleased with the choice they made and outcome that resulted.

Q. What are the main benefits of choosing Invisalign over other tooth alignment options?

A. This is a question that if not being asked, should be asked. The benefits of the Invisalign System are what make it so incredible! There are a variety of benefits that are provided, which we have gone over quite a bit in detail throughout prior chapters. The main benefits of Invisalign include:

- **Technology.** Because the Invisalign System uses such advanced technology, it is able to provide a precise treatment plan and predictable outcome. The technology that drives the system allows the doctor to help plan and even show the patient what the outcome will look like. It's a treatment plan that is customizable and even allows for changes along the way.

- **Invisibility.** One of the greatest things about Invisalign is that it has been designed to be nearly invisible and provide people with a discreet treatment option. With Invisalign, you can forget having to flash a mouth of metal every time you speak or smile. The majority of people will never even know that you are undergoing treatment, at least unless you bring it to their attention.

- **Hygiene.** As we have discussed prior, maintaining good oral hygiene is essential to overall health and wellness. Unlike other tooth alignment options, such as metal or ceramic braces, Invisalign allows you to remove the aligners in order to maintain proper brushing and flossing habits during treatment.

- **Flexibility.** With metal and ceramic braces, you have no ability to remove them during treatment. So if they are bothering you and you just want to take a break, or you have a day where you want to have some sticky taffy, you have no options. With Invisalign, you have the ability to remove the aligner! So there is no need to pass up on that caramel apple that you usually have each fall. Just remove your aligner and enjoy!

- **Comfort.** In addition to Invisalign providing more social comfort and confidence, it is also a more comfortable system all the way around. Rather than having wires and brackets poking your mouth, you will have smooth aligners that should not irritate your mouth. Invisalign makes tooth alignment more comfortable than ever before.

- **Shorter treatment time.** Those who choose Invisalign will typically have a treatment plan spanning the course of a year. Compare that to the two or more years that someone might wear metal or ceramic braces. Not only is the treatment time shorter, but you will also spend less time in the doctor's chair and go for fewer appointments over the course of the treatment.

Q. Is the Invisalign treatment system painful?

A. If you are an adult, you may recall a time when your classmates had a rough day due to their braces. They may have been in pain, trying various things to alleviate it, or even checking out early to head to the doctor's office to seek comfort. Truth be told, metal braces, while having had a place in our history, did cause people quite a bit of discomfort. Invisalign largely takes care of the discomfort issue.

With braces, discomfort can be an ongoing concern. For patients with Invisalign, it is not a big issue. Most people tend to experience mild discomfort for the first week that they begin treatment. It's not a lot of pain or anything, but it does take a few days to get used to wearing an aligner on their teeth. Once you have adjusted to the treatment, there is minimal discomfort. Some people have complained of slight discomfort each time they begin a new aligner, typically for 1-2 days.

Each time you begin a new aligner, it may take you a day to really feel comfortable in it, but you should not experience significant pain. The discomfort with Invisalign should be minimal, if at all. Think of getting Invisalign like getting a new pair of shoes. After a few days it will be like you've always had them.

Q. How often do I change the aligners with Invisalign?

The treatment process with the Invisalign System typically calls for about a year-long plan. Throughout treatment you can expect to change aligners, or "trays," every two weeks. Changing aligners allows your treatment to progress to the next stage. Each new aligner represents the next step in your treatment.

The fact that you get to change your aligners every two weeks will keep you motivated. You will see that you are continuously making progress toward reaching your end goal of having straight teeth. Before you know it, the year will have gone by, and you will have a brand new smile to show the world.

Q. Will the Invisalign aligners leave stains or marks on my teeth as some braces do?

A. One of the many benefits of using Invisalign is that they will not stain or leave any marks on your tooth. In fact, many people choose to go with bleaching their teeth at some point in the treatment process, since they already have a custom fitted tray.

If you would like to have your teeth whitened, discuss this option with your orthodontist. Some may prefer to do it before or at the end of the treatment, but you should be able to finish your treatment with not only a smile featuring straight teeth, but one featuring whiter teeth as well.

Q. How long do I need to wear each aligner during the day?

A. Align Technology recommends that you wear your aligners 20 to 22 hours per day. Most orthodontists will recommend wearing them 22 hours per day. This is just to maximize the effectiveness. I personally recommend to my patients to also shoot for wearing them at least 22 hours per day. This still provides plenty of time for removing them for brushing, flossing, eating, or other special occasions.

Q. Why do people choose to engage in tooth alignment, especially if they are already an adult?

A. There are millions of adults who look in the mirror everyday and wish the smile looking back at them was different. They long for straighter teeth. This is often one of the main reasons that people seek tooth alignment. Common reasons for needing Invisalign include crowded teeth, spacing issues, and bites that are misaligned.

Doctors also recommend Invisalign for overall oral health. As you have previously learned throughout this book, misaligned teeth can lead to oral health issues because they are more difficult to brush and floss properly.

No matter what the reason for straightening your teeth, whether for health or aesthetics, there are plenty of valuable reasons and benefits for making the choice to avoid living with crooked teeth. Millions of people who have gone through the process are happy that they did.

My guess is that it would be difficult to find people who now have straight teeth, as a result of undergoing Invisalign, who regret having made the decision to have the treatment. But you will always find people well into their adulthood who wish they had undergone treatment to straighten their teeth. Choosing to straighten your teeth has many benefits and leaves you with no regrets!

Q. What is interproximal enamel reduction?

A. If you have crowded teeth, there is a chance that your doctor will recommend interproximal enamel reduction. It sounds kind of confusing if you are not familiar with it, but it is much simpler than it sounds. Interproximal enamel reduction reduces the size of the enamel on the teeth that are crowded.

This procedure is often performed if you have crowded teeth in order to increase the effectiveness of your alignment treatment. If your teeth are crowded and you do not have the interproximal enamel reduction performed, you may not have as much success with alignment.

This is a safe procedure that is performed by your doctor prior to beginning specific phases of wearing aligners. This is just one more reason that you should opt for an orthodontic specialist. The orthodontist has the necessary expertise and education to perform the procedure accurately and precisely.

Q. Does it matter if I choose an orthodontist or a dentist?

A. If your car needed new tires, would you prefer to take it to a place that specialized in tires or one that was a general garage, providing all types of services on your vehicle? Chances are, you would rather take it to a tire specialist. After all, they probably know more about tires, have had more experience with them, and likely have more options available from which to choose. They are, after all, experts in their field.

The same goes for choosing a dentist or an orthodontist when it comes to tooth alignment. A dentist has been trained on the overall care of your teeth, but they are not a specialist in any one area. Many of their days are spent providing check-ups and dental fillings. But it's different with orthodontists.

An orthodontist is a specialist at tooth alignment. To become an orthodontist, one has to attend and graduate from dental school, but they have to go beyond that and complete 2-3 years of study that focus only on straightening the teeth and jaws.

In other words, an orthodontist is a specialist in the exact area that you are interested in, straightening your teeth, so the question becomes why would you ever want to go elsewhere? By choosing an orthodontist to straighten your teeth, you are choosing an expert who spends their days doing exactly that. Orthodontists have the knowledge, experience, and expertise to help you successfully achieve your tooth alignment goals.

Q. How many sets of Invisalign trays will I go through during my treatment?

A. The number of different trays that you will use in your treatment depends on your individual and customized plan. Everyone is different, so there's no set number of trays. This is something that will be determined between your doctor and those working in the Align Technology lab, as they work together to create the best possible treatment for your individual goals.

The average length of time that the Invisalign treatment takes is around one year. Considering you change aligners to progress to the next treatment phase, every two weeks, you can expect to go through roughly 25-26 sets of aligners. You will stop in at your doctor's office to pick up new trays every 6-12 weeks. Along the way they will ensure everything is going as planned.

One of the unique benefits of Invisalign is that changes to your treatment plan can be made at any time during the treatment process. So if you stop in and the doctor sees something that needs to be adjusted, it can be done in order to keep you on track for a successful tooth alignment outcome.

Q. How does the Invisalign System work to straighten my teeth?

A. The advanced technology that Align Technology has created with the Invisalign System aligns your teeth by using a series of thermoplastic trays, or aligners. In the beginning of your treatment, a plan will be mapped out, and the treatment will consist of you changing your aligner every two weeks. Each aligner progresses your treatment to the next phase, moving your teeth a little bit at a time, until they are finally in the desired position by the time you are finished with your final set of aligners.

Invisalign offers a customizable treatment, so each person's plan that is mapped out for treatment varies. Some trays might move a tooth as precisely as one-tenth of one millimeter before the next aligner picks up where that tray left off and continues the treatment. Their system is precise and offers excellent results!

Q. How often will I need to have an appointment with my doctor?

A. Invisalign patients can plan on seeing their doctor about every six to 12 weeks. This gives the doctor the opportunity to check on the progress of the treatment and ensure everything is going according to the plan that was created.

This is a great time for you to ask questions and bring up any type of issues or concerns you may have. If the doctor feels there are adjustments that need to be made to your treatment plan, they will be discussed at this time and planned into the overall outcome.

Q. Will wearing the Invisalign trays impair my speech?

A. Anytime you wear a dental appliance you may find that there is a temporary change or impact in your speech. The same goes with the aligners. But this is just temporary, and as soon as your tongue gets used to the aligners being in your mouth, you should not have any speech issues. Most people who experience a slight lisp or speech issues only do so for the first day or two of treatment. If your lisp continues beyond one to two days, ask your orthodontist for suggestions to help your tongue adapt more quickly.

Q. How will Invisalign impact my eating habits?

A. As you are finding out, there are many great benefits of Invisalign for teeth straightening. One of them is that it has no impact on your food choices or how you eat. A requirement of wearing the aligners is that you have to remove them to eat, so you have no restrictions on what you can and cannot eat. Each time you go to eat, simply remove the aligners.

This is certainly different from wearing metal or ceramic braces, as both come with a list of food items that should not be eaten. If you do end up eating some of those things on the list, it can damage your braces and delay your treatment plan. This is just one more reason that Invisalign makes treatment much more comfortable and convenient.

Q. Will I be able to smoke during my Invisalign treatment?

A. If you smoke while having your aligners in your mouth, there is a good chance you will stain them. Smoking stains your teeth, and will end up doing the same to the aligners. It's best to avoid smoking while using Invisalign. This may be a good time to kick the habit or seek alternatives during treatment. Some people choose to simply remove their aligner each time they smoke, but your doctor's overall recommendation for oral health will include smoking cessation.

Q. *How do you clean Invisalign trays?*

A. The best way to keep your trays clean is to use the Invisalign cleaning kit that you will get when you start treatment. You can also brush them and rinse with warm water to keep them clean. Remove the trays for all foods and any liquids other than water. Following these rules will keep your trays sparkling clean.

Q. *I have had special dental work or braces, so can I still get Invisalign?*

A. There are some people who would like Invisalign to straighten their teeth, but they may have had certain types of dental work in the past. Some people have already had braces and their teeth have shifted, while others may have veneers or bridges. If you fall into this category and are interested in Invisalign, you will need to meet with an orthodontist to discuss your options. Sometimes Invisalign, compared to braces and metal wires, is your best option to straighten teeth with large fillings or crowns, so it is worth asking your orthodontist.

Q. What happens once I'm finished with my Invisalign treatment?

A. That is a question that doesn't have one straight answer. Some people may need a retainer that they wear at night, while others need a fixed retainer on the inside surface of their teeth. It all depends on your own treatment plan, which needs to be evaluated and discussed with your doctor. Consistent follow-up during the retainer phase of treatment is critical to your long-term success and healthy smile.

As you can see, there are many questions that people have regarding Invisalign. Hopefully, I have answered your questions here, and you feel that you have a good idea of what all is involved. If you have additional questions, you may find the answers in the coming chapters, or you can always contact an orthodontist for an expert opinion. Visit Braces.org to locate an orthodontic specialist in your area.

Invisalign, like any type of orthodontic treatment, comes with a variety of questions from the consumer. But the more you know, the more comfortable you will feel about the treatment and outcome!

"I've had 29 trays and also invested in professional tooth whitening. I am officially done with the treatment, and I must say that it was all money well worth spending."

-Julie, New York

CHAPTER SIX:
So, you've decided to start Invisalign. Now what?

At this point you may have already decided that Invisalign is right for you. Great! But you still may not be sure what comes next. Just making the decision to start the treatment doesn't always mean you know the next steps in the process. That's where this chapter comes in.

Throughout this chapter, we will look at how you can get started and what you can expect once you get your first set of Invisalign trays. After you complete this chapter, you will have a good idea of how the process gets started and what those first weeks of treatment will be like.

Getting Started

Your first step in starting the Invisalign treatment is to visit with the orthodontist, if you haven't already done that. As you read this, you may have already had an initial consultation with an orthodontist to see if you are a good candidate for

Invisalign. If you haven't, now is the time to make an appointment to do so.

After you meet with the orthodontist to discuss if you are a good candidate for Invisalign, you will move on to the phase where your individual treatment plan is designed to meet your specific alignment goals. As you may recall from prior chapters, this process involves having x-trays and impressions taken of your mouth and teeth. The information will be gathered and put into the computer program so that a plan can be created to help you meet your alignment needs.

Once the information is collected and recorded, it will be sent to Align Technology, where your first aligners will be created. Within about two weeks, you will have your first set of aligners and be ready to meet with the doctor in order to officially get the treatment phase started.

Next, I am going to break down the Invisalign process in a series of weeks. This will give you a good idea what to expect during the first month, as opposed to the rest of the treatment, and even what to expect after the initial treatment has been completed.

Receiving Your First Trays

Finally, the day has arrived that you get to stop by the doctor's office and pick up your first set of Invisalign trays. You have been anticipating this day for quite a while and it has finally arrived. As you meet with the doctor, be prepared to ask any questions you may have. If you need to, write them down and take the list of questions along with you.

When you walk out of the doctor's office that first day, you want to be confident that you know what you are doing and that you do not have questions that you forgot to ask. Not that you can't still get them answered or place a call to the doctor's office, but you will just feel better, and more confident, having had your questions answered prior to leaving.

With your first set of aligner trays, you will also get a kit that comes with cleaning instructions and some other helpful things. This will get you started in knowing how to remove and clean the trays, but you may still likely have questions, as many people do, which is perfectly normal.

As you know, your treatment will consist of a series of Invisalign aligner trays that will move the teeth into place throughout the course of the treatment plan. Every two weeks you will have a new set of trays, which works to advance the treatment another step closer to completion.

Weeks One Through Four

Once you get your first set of trays, there are some things you will experience that you should be aware of. The more you are aware of them, the more you will be ready to address them, or realize that they are only temporary conditions. And even though there are some issues you may experience with your Invisalign trays, keep in mind that any tooth alignment option you choose is going to have some issues that arise.

There is no way to align the teeth without having some mild discomfort or irritation during the first one to two days. With Invisalign, however, most people seem to find that there are fewer issues than with braces, including less pain and discomfort. Having said that, there are a few issues that may arise, causing you minimal discomfort when you get started with your Invisalign trays. Not everyone experiences these issues, but if you are aware of their risks in advance, you can be prepared.

Here are some of the issues that may come up in the first four weeks of wearing your Invisalign aligners:

- **Planning your appointments.** It is important that you plan appointments that will work around your schedule. You will be going to the doctor's every six to twelve weeks to pick up new aligners. Be sure to book your appointments at a time that will be convenient for you. Your doctor will most likely be happy to work with you to ensure it is convenient and fits into your schedule.

- **Cheek or tongue soreness**. Some people do find that they experience some minor cheek or tongue soreness during the first week that they start wearing their aligners. It is not usually major or anything to worry about, but if you do experience some minor discomfort, know that it is perfectly normal and that it should go away within a few days. The first week that people start the treatment and wear the aligners is the most challenging because it takes your mouth time to get used to having something new. You will get used to it within a week, and this cheek and tongue soreness will naturally subside. If you find you have soreness, try using a warm saltwater rinse and an over-the-counter pain reliever, such as Advil, to help alleviate the discomfort. Typically any pain or discomfort that people feel during this first week of adjustment is minor and temporary. It may just be more annoying to you during the first week than painful, as you adjust to having something new in your mouth and on your teeth. But you will adjust, as everyone else does, so just be patient the first week or so as you allow your mouth to get used to having aligners.

- **Tooth soreness or sensitivity.** When you first begin wearing aligners, you may find that your teeth feel a bit sensitive to hot, cold, or pressure. This is normal and like other discomfort issues will go away after you adjust, which may take a week or so. If your teeth do feel sensitive, you may want to account for that during this time by avoiding foods that are really crunchy, for example. Over the counter pain relievers like Advil are recommended during the first day or two to help alleviate any discomfort.

- **Talking with a lisp.** For the first few days that you begin to wear your aligners, you may find that you talk with a lisp or that your speech doesn't sound as it usually does. A lisp is usually noticeable when pronouncing "s" or "z" words. When it happens as a result to beginning to wear Invisalign trays, it is because your tongue is not used to the trays. As you speak more, your tongue will adjust to the aligners and your speech should go back to normal. One thing you can do to help get past the lisp quicker is to sing as you are driving around in the car. This will help your tongue get used to the aligners faster, which will get you past the lisp faster. Some people never experience a lisp, and others feel they have it longer than the first week. However, it is often something you may hear, or believe you hear, while others do not detect it when you are speaking. In other words, you may be more sensitive to picking it up than other people who are listening to you. For the majority of people who wear Invisalign, the lisp during the first week, as they adjust, is not a big issue.

- **Putting in the aligners and removing them**. Most people tend to have a learning curve when it comes to learning how to easily remove their Invisalign aligners. Like most things, with practice you will get better. In order for the aligners to do their job of straightening your teeth, they must fit tightly. They are doing their job if they fit your teeth snuggly. But this snugness may also make it a little more challenging for someone to remove their aligners if they are new to wearing them. The best thing to do is relax, be patient, and practice. By the time you are ready for your second set of aligners, two weeks later, you should no longer have difficulty removing them. The difficulty in the beginning only happens because it is something new, and you need to practice. By the time you reach the half way mark of your treatment, you will be popping them out without even thinking about it and wondering why you had so much trouble to begin with.

There are a few other things that you will want to keep in mind during this initial stage as well. For starters, some people find that they tend to snack less throughout the day. This is because they don't want to remove the aligners. You absolutely can remove them to snack, but some patients have reported that they tend to snack less, which for many people turns out to be a good side effect of having the aligners on.

If you wish to snack less, great, but don't feel you have to on the account of the aligners. As long as you are wearing your aligners for the recommended time per day, of at least 22 hours per day, it is perfectly fine to remove them for meals, snacks, brushing, etc. just remember to brush or rinse your mouth out with water prior to placing the aligners back on your teeth.

Adjustment Period

No matter what age you are right now, you have most likely lived this far without aligners in your mouth. The way your mouth is right now is what you are used to. If you have ever gone to the dentist and had any work done, such as a crown or filling, you know that when the dentist is done and the anesthetic wears off, your mouth feels a little different for a while.

It may take you a few days to get used to the new way your mouth or tooth feels. During that time, you may run your tongue over your tooth often, feeling the new way that it feels. This is similar to how your transition is going to be to wearing Invisalign trays.

Your first week or so of wearing the trays is going to be an adjustment period. During this time, you will likely feel them a lot with your tongue, view them a lot in the mirror, and spend time getting used to the way they feel. You will also spend time getting to know how it feels to talk with them, as well as remove them, and keep them clean.

It's important to realize that there is an adjustment period just as there is with anything else. So go into your treatment knowing that the first week will be a learning curve, as well as an adjustment period. But know that you will learn it, as you do everything else, and you will adjust. Before you know it, the aligners will be old news, and you will just turn your focus on completing the treatment so that you can enjoy an amazing smile!

Week Five and Beyond

By the time you get to this point, you will be used to your new aligners and will be focused on advancing your treatment. Every two weeks you will change aligners as you continue to move forward. Each time you go to your doctor's office, feel free to ask any questions you may have, as well as bring up any concerns.

Each time you get new aligners, it may take you a day or so to get used to them. They will feel a little bit different than the ones did before, including feeling tighter. As mentioned before, the tightness is necessary to further the treatment and move the teeth into position.

Although there is a small adjustment period when starting a new set of trays, most people adjust within a day of getting them. If your adjustment period takes longer than that or there seems to be issues that you find extremely bothersome, contact your doctor to discuss the issue and see what can be done.

From week five through the end of your treatment, you can expect to continue the process getting new aligners as scheduled. You will need to be sure to clean them, following the instructions you receive from your doctor, and continue your good brushing and flossing habits. The treatment will go by quicker than you may realize, as it does for most people.

Tips and Tricks for Success

Just telling you to wear your aligners is not enough to ensure that everything goes smoothly, and you remain happy throughout the process. There are some tips and tricks for success that you can keep in mind. By implementing some, if not all, of these practices, you can help to make your treatment period smoother, as well as more successful.

- **Missed appointments.** If you miss an appointment, be sure to contact your doctor. You will need to make sure that you schedule another one promptly. This is especially important if it is time to get the next set of aligners. Delaying an appointment once, or for a day, will not cause problems. But if you continuously miss appointments and delay moving to the next set of aligners, you could be delaying your treatment. The only way that the orthodontist can be sure that your treatment is progressing is by seeing you consistently at each appointment. Your appointments with the doctor are a crucial part of the treatment process that helps to ensure a successful outcome.

- **Not wearing trays 22 hours per day.** One of the benefits of wearing Invisalign trays, as you have already been made aware, is the fact that you can remove them. Treatment options such as braces don't offer such convenience. However, being able to remove them any time you'd like means that you have to be disciplined. While it may be tempting to remove them often, you have to avoid doing this for the sake of a successful treatment outcome. It is important that you make the commitment to wearing your aligners for at least 22 hours per day. If you take them out more frequently, you may set back your treatment, as you will not be progressing as planned. So while you can take them out for a total of up to two hours per day, be sure to make it a point to wear them for 22 hours each day. The two hours per day that you can remove your Invisalign aligners is going to likely end up being used for eating, brushing and flossing, and other such activities. The Invisalign System will only work while you are actually wearing your aligners, so it is essential to keep them in for at least the 22 hours per day.

- **Not forgetting your aligners.** While this is not common, there are some people that tend to forget about their aligners when they first start wearing them and take them out to eat in a restaurant. If you are dining out and remove them to eat, don't forget them on your plate or in your napkin and have them whisked away when the table is cleared. Be sure to pay attention to where they are; keep tabs of them once you are done eating.

- **Keep teeth together.** As previously mentioned, each time you start a new set of aligners, you will find that it takes a day or so to get used to them. You can help to speed up this process by keeping your teeth together, yet not in a clenching state, which will help to speed up the fit and efficiency process of the treatment.

- **Seeing the dentist.** As you are probably aware, it is recommended that you see your dentist every six months for a check-up and/or cleaning. You will likely be wearing your aligners during the time that you should be seeing your dentist. While you might be thinking you can skip the appointment since you are undergoing treatment, my recommendation is that you continue to see your dentist every four to six months during treatment. As you have already read in an earlier chapter, it is important to maintain good oral hygiene, so you should continue to visit the dentist. Just be sure to let them know, if the doctor doesn't already, that you are currently wearing Invisalign aligners and offer the name of your orthodontist, just in case there are any questions. Having said that, it is important that you meet with your dentist prior to Invisalign treatment, so you can have any issues addressed before to starting initial treatment and having impressions taken. This way there will not be changes in the impressions and information gathered about your teeth should you need a cavity filled or tooth repair.

- **Progress x-rays.** You may find that from time to time your orthodontist would like you to get x-rays. This is to check on your progress and ensure that the treatment is going according to plan.

- **Mid-course corrections.** Throughout the course of treatment, some patients might need a mid-course correction. This is when the original treatment plan must be re-planned in order to compensate for some changes that have taken place with your mouth or teeth. This may happen as a result of you having some dental work, such as fillings, or from some type of trauma that has occurred. If this does happen, it requires additional work in creating a new treatment plan, so there is usually a one to two week work-up by your doctor before receiving your corrected aligners.

- **Store them correctly.** When you get your aligners, you will be given a storage case. Be sure to always store them properly when you are not wearing them so that you don't lose or damage them. If you do lose them, you will incur a charge for each replacement aligner. Avoid storing your aligners in the car during hot summer months and do not place them in boiling water to disinfect them after a cold or a flu virus. Heat will damage and distort your aligners, making them ineffective if able to be worn at all.

- **Maintain order.** Although you realize you will switch aligners every two weeks, it is important to make sure you are wearing them in the correct sequential order to help ensure your treatment success. Each stage of aligners has been carefully planned to move your teeth to the next stage of the treatment. Look on the biting surface of the back molar teeth for the number of your current tray. Your second tray will say "02N".

- **Aligner spacing.** It is important that your current aligners fit without any spaces before you go onto the next aligner. If you find that there are spaces between your teeth and the aligner, you should continue wearing it for a few more days until there are no spaces, and then move on to the next aligner. Speak with your orthodontist about this to confirm whether he or she suggests you wear your aligners longer if you still have spaces.

- **Keeping old aligners.** Ideally you should keep your last three sets of aligners. This is ideal because if you lose one or there is an aligner that does not fit, you will be able to go back in sequence and then catch up when the new fitted one arrives.

- **Hygiene aides.** While your Invisalign aligners will come with a basic kit, there are some additional hygiene aides that you can use. Align Technology, for example, offers an additional cleaning system for purchase, which comes with cleaning crystals. They have been designed to give your aligners the cleaning that they need and should have on a regular basis. If you need additional hygiene aides beyond your toothbrush and floss for getting your teeth clean, consider such options as inter-dental cleaners, mouth rinses, oral irrigators, rubber tip simulators, and even tongue cleaners. If you need recommendations, don't hesitate to speak with your orthodontist or dentist, who may also have product samples for you to try out before making purchases.

After Invisalign Treatment

No matter how short or long your Invisalign treatment process is, there will come a time when you have reached the end. This is the day you have waited for! You will get to see your new smile and show it off to everyone.

Just as knowing what to expect before and during treatment is beneficial, knowing what to expect once the active treatment phase has reached completion is helpful as well.

If you recall from prior chapters, when you get started with Invisalign, your treatment plan consists of phases. Each of these phases, which last around two weeks each, will progress your treatment toward the final goal. Once you reach the end of that plan, there is usually some finishing work that needs to be done in order to help maintain the investment that you have made into your new smile.

Once you finish the process of wearing the Invisalign aligners, you may need to have refinements (or final detailing of your bite) made, or may even need several additional aligners that were not initially planned. This is done to provide the finishing touches, so to speak, to the treatment. Rarely, some patients also need to wear a few clear braces in order to help finish the treatment successfully.

After you have completed treatment, include additional aligners if needed, you will then begin to wear a clear retainer. The clear retainer is generally worn all the time for around six months, and then after that you will just continue to wear it to bed. Wearing this retainer helps to ensure that your treatment remains successful. It's a simple way to help protect the investment you made in your new smile.

Once you have completed the six months of wearing a retainer full time after completing the aligner phases, you will only be wearing a retainer while sleeping. During the day, you will have nothing but a new beautiful smile!

Some patients may find that they need to have braces on one or two teeth following treatment. While this is not common, the possibility does exist, depending on your treatment needs and the initial outcome. This is an issue that you would need to speak to your orthodontist about, but if it is necessary, it is just one more step in the process of ensuring that your alignment finishes perfectly.

Getting Started

When you have made the decision to get started with Invisalign, simply give your orthodontist a call. The sooner you get started, the sooner you will be on your way to a smile that you have always wanted and the tooth alignment that you should have.

The path to straight teeth is just around the corner. To get there, all you need to do is make the first step and meet with the orthodontist to get the process started. You will be glad you did!

> *"My one piece of advice for anyone that uses Invisalign is that you never lose sight of them! Being able to remove them to eat is wonderful, but don't make the mistake I made. I wrapped it up in a napkin, left it on the plate, and never saw it again. Keeping track of it at all times is crucial!"*
>
> *–Lisa, Michigan*

CHAPTER SEVEN:
Who else is a good candidate for Invisalign?

If you have been reading this book thinking about Invisalign for yourself, you already have an idea of whether or not the treatment is right for you. But many people may be reading this book in an effort to determine if Invisalign is ideal for other family members, such as their teenage children.

In this chapter, we are going to take a look at who else Invisalign may be a good option for, such as teenagers. We will also take a look at when Invisalign may not be the best option for some patients.

Invisalign Teen

At this point, you have learned a great deal about Invisalign. But what you may not be aware of is that Invisalign Teen has been designed to meet the growing needs of the teenager, while providing the necessary teeth straightening as effectively as braces do.

The reasons why a teen would want to get Invisalign over other braces are the same for adults. Yet there reasoning may even be more pronounced because as we know, kids can be brutal.

Today there is a lot of bullying and teasing that goes on at schools. We have always had bullying and teasing, but it seems that in recent years it has become more out of control. Teens who wear braces may feel that they are going to be targeted for teasing. This may not always happen, but most teens find that they feel more confident if they are not wearing metal braces.

Teens who get Invisalign can carry on with their normal schedules, which may include school, work, and social activities, without having to worry about their smile. They can silently wear Invisalign to treat their misaligned teeth but will not have to lose self confidence or shy away from activities because they worry about their smile.

With Invisalign Teen, your teen will their teeth straightened with nearly invisible aligners. Their treatment will likely be around a year long, and they can go about their normal brushing, flossing, and eating, just like they did before orthodontic treatment.

The Blue Dot

Every Invisalign Teen aligner comes with a small Blue Dot Wear Indicator, which is quite inconspicuous. This indicator, sometimes referred to as a compliance indicator, helps your teen know how long they have been wearing each aligner and when it is time to swap them out for the next pair, thus advancing the treatment.

With Invisalign Teen, your teen can have the benefits of avoiding the pain and discomfort that comes with wearing metal braces. They will also be able to take them out for their school pictures or other short functions. Plus, kids like to eat a lot of things like gummy candies, popcorn, apples, corn on the cob, carrots, bagels, pizza crust, and even pretzels and nuts that would likely be off limits if they were wearing braces. While some adults may not mind forgoing all of these foods for one or two years during treatment, there are many teens that will find it extremely difficult.

If your teen has metal braces and decides to eat these foods, they may cause damage to the brackets, which will lead to a quick trip to the orthodontist, along with some pain and discomfort until the repairs are made. Broken braces also cause delays on treatment and additional time out of school or other activities.

With Invisalign, your teen doesn't have to give up any of these foods. They can eat what they want, when they want it. All they need to do is simply remove the aligners while they eat. Plus, the Invisalign aligners will not irritate their gums or their mouth. It has a smooth feeling that has been designed to avoid the irritations caused by metal braces and wires.

Invisalign gives your teen the ability to go about their life, not making big sacrifices, like they would with traditional braces. They can enjoy their normal activities, foods, and hygiene habits, without making sacrifices.

Invisalign Teen vs. Braces

Invisalign Teen	Braces
Nearly invisible treatment.	Noticeable treatment.
Can be removed to eat, drink and perform dental hygiene routine.	Cannot be removed during treatment.
No pain from broken brackets or wires.	Will likely experience some pain from broken wires and brackets.
Less frequent visits to see the doctor.	More frequent visits to see the doctor due to routine appointments and broken hardware.
Can be removed to eat foods, such as gummy candy, popcorn, apples, etc.	Cannot be removed to eat at all.
Typical treatment time of one year.	Treatment may take several years to complete.
Uses advanced software that allows the patient to see in advance what the results will look like.	Does not have as advanced software to help provide a look at what the outcome will be.
Is made from smooth, clear, comfortable plastic	Is made from wires & brackets, which may break & poke into the mouth.
A highly precise and customizable solution.	Standard appliance. One size fits all.
Aligners can be removed & cleaned.	
Provides 6 free aligner replacements for those that are lost or damaged.	

Additional Perks

With Invisalign Teen there are additional perks, such as not having as many appointments to attend. Teens today have a schedule each week that is filled with activities. From school and work to sporting activities and everything in between, they already have a full schedule.

Invisalign Teen is going to help keep your teen out of the orthodontist chair more than if they have metal braces. With metal braces, there will be more doctor visits and longer appointments at each visit, which will require more juggling of their already busy schedule.

Many parents find that having fewer appointments for their teen to attend is beneficial. That way they don't have to miss any of the other commitments that they already have planned. Invisalign Teen saves you, and your teen, a lot of time that would otherwise be spent visiting the orthodontist.

With Invisalign Teen, there is an additional perk that is not offered to adults. They are allowed to have up to five free replacement aligners, should they lose or break one. Usually replacing missing or damaged aligners takes just a couple of days at the most.

This is an important benefit because as we know, teens may be a little harder on and less watchful of their aligners than adults are. So if they lose them, or happen to break them, you can rest assured knowing that they your teen will be able to get up to five aligners replaced for no additional cost.

Considering Alternatives

Some parents inquire about getting veneers for their teen, or themselves, in an effort to improve the appearance of the teeth. Veneers absolutely have their place in the world of orthodontics and dentistry, but using them in place of Invisalign Teen is not usually the best option.

Most orthodontists will not do veneers on a teenager because of the risk that they are still growing. So for teenagers, veneers are not usually a recommended alternative. Even for adults, as we have discussed previously, they are not always the best route to take.

How Invisalign Teen Works

Invisalign Teen works the same way that the aligner system works for adults. So everything that you have read so far in previous chapters stands true for teens as well. The good news for teens is that you can also get the Invisalign Teen system while teeth are still growing.

Your teen can also get Invisalign even if all their permanent teeth have yet to come in. In fact, the Invisalign Teen has been designed to meet the needs of a growing teen and things like erupting molars have been accounted for and will not deter the treatment at all.

The Invisalign teen aligners have been designed to have "eruption tabs" to account for the person's erupting second molars. In addition to this, the system also has "power ridges" that have been designed to help meet the needs of successfully moving those teeth that may be seen, historically, as difficult movements.

With a treatment time of about a year, Invisalign Teen will help your teen to have straighter teeth, without all the sacrifice. Within a year, they will have a straight, beautiful smile. Maybe even just in time for their senior pictures.

The Invisalign Teen system works in the same way that the adult system does. So once the images and molds are taken of the teeth, the aligners will be custom made. Then your teen will begin wearing a new set of aligners every two weeks. With each set of new aligners, their teeth will be advancing to the next stage of the treatment.

The blue dot helps teens to determine that it is time to move onto the next set, as it will turn clear once they have reached the two week mark. This is only going to happen if they wear them the recommended time each day, which I recommend to be around 22 hours per day. So if your teen wants to keep removing them more than the recommended amount of time each day, the blue dot will not turn clear at the two-week mark, indicating they are not ready to go on to the next set of aligners and advance their treatment.

It's important to note that the blue dot is in the back of the mouth on one of the last teeth. So there is no worrying about people being able to see it. Even with the blue dot on the aligner, your teen's tooth alignment will still be nearly invisible. It's usually not visible by others when you have the aligner on your teeth.

It is important that your teen understands they will need to wear the aligners for at least 22 hours per day, in order for their treatment to be successful and not be delayed. If they do not, they may have to extend the time that they wear their aligner trays, or their total treatment time may be extended.

Although your teen can expect to change their aligners every two weeks, they will only be meeting with the doctor every six to twelve weeks. So this gives you an idea of the time involved and the commitment that will be needed on their part, as well as on yours if you will be providing the transportation.

Why the Blue Dot

The reason the blue dot was added to the teen model of Invisalign is that many parents are often concerned that their teen might remove the aligners for longer than the recommended period of time. With the blue dot, there is no guessing as to whether or not your teen is ready to move onto the next level of aligners. The blue dot speaks for itself in letting the wearer, as well as the doctor, know if they have been wearing them according to the instructions and are ready or if they need to wear the aligners a little longer. The blue compliance indicator, therefore, is great for peace of mind and knowing that your teen is wearing the aligners for the recommended 22 hours per day.

Reasons for Invisalign Teen

The reasons that teens might get Invisalign are the same reasons that adults do. There are many benefits to having straight teeth. Here are some of the specific reasons that teens would seek Invisalign treatment:

- Fixing an overbite or underbite.

- Fixing a spacing or crowding issue.

- Straightening teeth in general.

- Seeking the perfect smile.

- To make a better first impression.

- To be more confident around others.

- For all the benefits that braces cannot provide.

Not only will Invisalign Teen take care of any spacing, crowding or alignment issues, but it will also help your teen feel more confident in life. When you have a nice smile, you feel good about showing it. When you have teeth that have an underbite or overbite or your teeth are crooked or crowded, you usually do not feel good and confident about smiling and talking with others.

Invisalign and Age Requirements

If you are considering Invisalign for your child, you may be wondering what age requirements there are. While there are no set rules about how old one needs to be in order to use the Invisalign treatment, most orthodontists would agree that somewhere around the age of 13 to 15 would be the minimum.

Some 13 year olds may be good candidates for Invisalign, but that all depends on their individual situation. Because of this, it is important to meet with an orthodontist and discuss whether or not it is the right route for your teen. Those who are 15 and up are usually good candidates for Invisalign treatment, unless there are other underlying issues, which we will discuss later in this chapter.

Additional Invisalign Plans

Along with the regular Invisalign plan and the Invisalign Teen plan, there are a couple of others that should be noted. Here's a short recap of what each of their main treatment plans are and the purpose they serve:

- **Invisalign Express 10.** This is a program that works just like the full program, only is a shorter one. It's typically for people who need only minor alignment corrections. The treatment can usually be completed within six months. It allows for purchasing one refinement but does not allow for mid-course correction.

- **Invisalign Express 5.** This is a program for those with minor issues, such as mild spacing, crowding, or other orthodontic issues. While using the same Invisalign technology, the treatment takes about 2.5 months, includes one automated refinement for purchase, but does not allow for mid-course correction.

- **Invisalign Teen.** This program, as discussed in this chapter, has been designed for the growing teenager. Treatment takes 12 to 18 months, three refinements are included, and mid-course correction is available for a fee. It also includes five free replacement aligners for those that are lost or damaged.

- **Invisalign Full.** This is the full program that has been described in-depth throughout this book. It generally takes 6 to 12 months for the treatment, allows up to three refinements that are included, and allows for a mid-course correction for a fee.

BPA Free

One thing that we have not mentioned yet is the safety of the plastic that is used to make Invisalign aligners. Many people today understandably have concerns about BPA being in plastics. BPA, which stands for bisphenol A, is an industrial chemical. It has been used in millions of plastic products since the 1960s.

The problem with BPA is that the National Institutes of Health has advised that there could be some health concerns with the use of it. It is believed, although research is still being conducted on it, that it speeds up puberty, endocrine issues, and other such problems, much of which is not even yet known or understood.

The good news on this issue is that the aligners are not made out of plastic containing the BPA resin. So you will not have to worry about the possible health issues associated with plastics that do have BPA. The Invisalign aligners are completely BPA free.

When Invisalign is Not the Best Option

While most people seem to be good candidates for the Invisalign System, there are some special cases that would make it not ideal. If there are issues present that make Invisalign not the best treatment, your orthodontist will discuss other options and help you find an ideal solution to achieve the results you are looking for in terms of both aesthetics and health.

Those who have orthodontic problems such as jawbone or bone structure issues may not be a good candidate for Invisalign. The same holds true for those who have other issues with their mouth that may be structural problems. There are other issues that some people have cited for reasons that they were not good candidates for Invisalign.

Here are some of the issues that would make someone a poor candidate for Invisalign treatment:

- Structural issues with the jawbone, bones, or other areas of the mouth.

- Anyone who has severe problems or issues with their teeth or mouth.

- Those who are unable to wear the trays 22 hours a day.

- Those who have severely tipped teeth, including those who have molars that have shifted into spaces where there has been an extraction.

- Anyone who has a severe tongue thrust.

If you have one of these conditions, don't automatically assume that Invisalign will not be an option for you. The best thing you can do is to meet with an orthodontist to discuss your options. Some people may still qualify for the treatment, so it is best to inquire and find out for sure.

Every person is different, so every recommendation is going to be different. You won't know if your teen, or yourself, is a good candidate for Invisalign until you meet with an orthodontist to discuss your particular case.

Paying for Invisalign Teen

When it comes to paying for Invisalign for your teen, there are the same payment options as for adults. First, you will want to check with your insurance provider to see if they will cover any of the costs. Beyond that, you can apply for third party financing, use healthy savings funds, and save up a year before getting it.

Additionally, most orthodontists have a variety of programs and suggestions for helping you to find funding options. Many orthodontists offer in-house financing, allowing you to make payments throughout the treatment.

Don't let money stop you from getting the treatment that your teen needs. There are many programs out there to help you get the treatment that is needed. Where there is a will, there is a way. And the benefits of having a great smile and maintaining confidence throughout the process last a lifetime.

Making the Call

As you can see, there are many benefits of choosing Invisalign for your teen in order to straighten their teeth. With today's use of technological advances in the field of orthodontics, now is the time to avoid a mouth full of metal. Today, your teenager can fix their teeth in a practically invisible manner, so it doesn't impede their life or self-confidence.

If you are not sure if your teen is ready for Invisalign, or is a good candidate for it, don't hesitate to contact your orthodontist. That's what they are there for, and they should be happy to answer your questions. Discuss the options with your teen to see what they feel is the best option for them. Then discuss it with your orthodontist so that together you can all find the best treatment option for your family and your teenager.

Invisalign Teen has proven to be a beneficial and successful treatment program that many people use across the country.

Chances are, if you choose Invisalign for your teen, you will be glad you did!

> *"My teen went with Invisalign. Once we sat down and evaluated the benefits of it, especially over braces, it was an easy decision. We couldn't be happier with the results."*
>
> *–Brenda, Oklahoma*

CHAPTER EIGHT:
The Importance of Retention After Orthodontic Treatment

Once you or your teen is finished with your initial Invisalign treatment, you will need to follow up with retention. The process of retention will keep your beautiful smiling looking that way for many years to come. In this chapter, we will look at the issue of retention and wearing a retainer.

Wearing a retainer is something that you will need to do after your Invisalign treatment plan is completed. Throughout this chapter you will learn everything you need to know about retainers, including why you need them, what they are made of, and what you can expect when you start wearing them.

Vivera Retainers

When it comes to using a retainer following your Invisalign treatment, you will be introduced to the Vivera line of retainers. The good news here is that they are created by Align Technology, the creators of Invisalign, so it makes for a smooth transition from the treatment phase to maintenance and retention.

Vivera is created using the same advanced technology that is used for the Invisalign aligners. They use advanced fabrication technology in order to create a precise, smooth, and comfortable retainer that will keep your new beautiful smile looking amazing for many years to come!

Another benefit of the Vivera retainer system is that it is unique to each patient just as the Invisalign aligners are. The clear thermoplastic retainer is considered to be 30 percent stronger than other retainer materials, and they can be made for top and bottom arches, as well as the full mouth and molar-to-molar retention.

Over time, Align Technology will ship four sets of the retainers to you, so you get the most successful results from your investment in the Invisalign treatment system. Using the Vivera retainer system helps to ensure that your beautiful smile will be professionally and successfully maintained.

Easy Ordering

As you can see throughout reading this book, Align Technology has really streamlined the entire process of this treatment system. They have carried that organization over to the Vivera retainers, as well. Since they can capture your digital dental records, they can keep them on file for future use and ease of ordering new retainers. New retainers can be easily ordered at any ClinCheck treatment stage.

Pontic Options

If you have any missing teeth in either your top or bottom arch, the Vivera retainers will account for that. They do this with using what is called "pontics." A pontic is an artificial tooth on a dental bridge. So your retainer would be designed having a pontic, or artificial tooth, in the space that you are missing the tooth.

Pontics are important in retention because they provide a solution to address the dental spaces and help keep your neighboring teeth from shifting or collapsing due to the lack of support in that area.

What to Expect With Your Retainer

Hearing that you may need to wear a retainer may seem like a scary thing at first. But that's probably because you are not familiar with what they are and what they do. Once you take the mystery out of retainers, it is clear to see that retainers are simple devices that help to maintain your bite, as well as sometimes address other conditions. And, they are nothing to be afraid of!

What They Are

You may have seen people wearing a retainer before, but they are not all that noticeable. A retainer is a small device that is made out of clear plastic, rubber, or even metal. They are custom-made so that they only fit your teeth. They are part of a treatment plan that has likely been determined by your orthodontist.

Using retainers to help align teeth is a common option. The length of time that someone has to wear them varies, but they are especially common following someone having their braces removed. During the process of wearing braces, the teeth have been moved into the desired position, but they are not yet settled into the gum and jaw.

By using a retainer, it helps to further set your teeth in their new position. Teeth tend to shift throughout your lifetime, so the retainer can help keep them where they are supposed to be until they are settled in and will not shift out of place.

Reasons for Wearing

The period of time immediately after the braces are removed is the most is when you are most likely to see your teeth shift. During this period of time (typically six months), the retainer is worn each day, and then you will wear it to bed at night for a while. This effort just helps to ensure that the new tooth placement is retained.

There are other conditions that call for a retainer as part of corrective treatment as well. Some of those conditions include:

- To close any small gaps that may be in the bite.

- To help correct speech problems in some patients.

- A variety of medical conditions, including tongue thrust, where the tongue goes between the teeth when talking and sleep apnea, where breathing is interrupted during sleep.

- To address bruxism, which is the grinding of the teeth while sleeping.

There are a variety of conditions that may call for a treatment plan that requires a retainer. Working with an orthodontist is the best way to determine if one can help with a particular condition and how long one would have to be worn, as the time varies depending on the severity of the problem being treated.

Preparing for a Retainer

When a retainer is being recommended as part of someone's treatment plan, it helps to know what to expect, such as a mold being made of your teeth. This is done with impression material called alginate, which makes a temporary mold of the teeth. That temporary mold is then used to make the retainer.

Retainers today have come a long way from the bigger pure metal ones of decades past. They can be customized to show your personality, including colors and pictures on them, or they can be clear plastic so that they are less noticeable to others. Depending on who is getting the retainer and their age, there are many options to consider.

Length, Care and Beyond

The length of time you can expect to wear your retainer varies. Much depends on the reason and severity of the treatment you are receiving. You can expect to meet with the orthodontist periodically, in order to make sure that everything is going according to the treatment plan and there is no discomfort.

Caring for a retainer is simple because it can easily be removed. It is recommended that they are cleaned daily, in order to maintain good oral hygiene and get rid of plaque and food particles. How the retainer is cleaned depends upon the type that you have, so you will need to check with the orthodontist for the cleaning recommendations on your specific version.

Retainers are part of a treatment plan that may address the misalignment of the teeth, closing gaps in the bite, correcting speech problems, and even assisting in medical conditions. Retainers are a simple device that can do an important job. Whether helping to get teeth settled in after braces, aligning teeth, or to correcting another condition, they are a treatment option that helps people to feel confident, as well as more comfortable.

More on Retainers

Years ago, orthodontists believed you could wear your retainers full time for a year or two and your teeth would stay straight for life. With today's research, however, we've discovered that teeth have the tendency to move and shift as you age. Crowding of the lower teeth is, in fact, a natural aging process. Therefore, the only way to guarantee your teeth stay straight for life is to wear your retainers (on some level) for life.

After the first 6 months of full-time retainer wear, night time retention is typically all that is needed in order to maintain your smile. Years after your Invisalign treatment is completed, you might wear your retainers 1-2 nights per week. If your teeth are straight and your retainers fit, there shouldn't be a problem maintaining your beautiful smile for life.

Factors Affecting Treatment Stability

Many of our patients ask what type of retainer we recommend. "Can I get a clear retainer?" or "will I need a fixed retainer?" are common patient questions. Your orthodontist takes into account several factors when he or she plans to retain the positions of your teeth. Growth of the jaws following treatment, the amount of time needed for gum and bone tissues to stabilize, and pressures from the lips and tongue are all important factors that affect the stability of your finished result. After considering these factors, your orthodontist decides what type of retainer you should wear and how long you should wear it.

Fixed Retainer

A fixed retainer is typically placed on the inside surfaces of the lower front teeth. This type of retainer can be attached to the two canine teeth or to every tooth in the area. A fixed retainer is very efficient at maintaining the positions of the teeth in certain situations. If your orthodontist decides to place a fixed retainer, it will make cleaning between your teeth more difficult.

Ask your orthodontist, dentist, and dental hygienist for tips and tricks to help you keep your teeth clean while wearing a fixed retainer. With proper care and regular visits to your general dentist, your fixed retainer can be left in place until lower jaw growth is completed (early adulthood) or indefinitely, as indicated.

Removable Retainers

Removable retainers have been used successfully for many years and are probably the most common type of retainer. Patients identify immediately with the wire that runs across the front teeth to help maintain tooth alignment and symmetry.

The Hawley retainer is probably the most popular type of removable retainer. It is made of plastic and stainless steel wire and is custom-made for your mouth and teeth. Variations of this type of retainer are too numerous to list, but they all achieve the same result – maintenance of your new smile for life.

Since removable retainers can be taken out, patients frequently ask how long they need to wear the retainer. Most relapse, or unwanted tooth movement, occurs in the first 3-6 months after the braces are removed. For the average patent, you will wear your removable retainer full-time for the first 3-6 months and thereafter only while sleeping.

If your orthodontist recommends a period of time longer or shorter than this, he or she is protecting your smile against the factors we mentioned at the beginning of the chapter. For example, a patient with severely misaligned jaws and teeth might wear retainers for a longer duration than a patient with only minor tooth-alignment problems.

If you are unsure of your retention program, be sure to ask your orthodontist or orthodontic assistant for specific instructions regarding the wear and care of your retainers.

Clear or Invisible Retainers

With the advent of new, clear plastic materials in orthodontics, patients can benefit from more aesthetic options during the retention phase of orthodontic treatment. Clear retainers are comfortable, aesthetic, and require no adjustment. However, they can be severely worn or broken if subjected to heavy biting forces. In our office, patients receive clear retainers as a back-up retainer and for social convenience during the first 3-6 months.

If the Hawley retainer is lost or broken, the clear retainer can be used as a back-up while our lab fabricates a new Hawley retainer. We have found this program to be very beneficial in maintaining healthy, beautiful smiles for life.

Retainer Wearing Tips

As you spend time wearing your retainer, you will end up coming across various questions. This is normal, so don't hesitate to call your doctor. Your retainer should always be comfortable; if you experience discomfort with your retainer, then it is a good time to give your orthodontist a call.

In this section I am going to go over some of the questions that frequently come up regarding retainers, covering some of the issues beyond what you have already read in the this chapter.

- **Bleaching teeth.** Many people want to know if they can bleach their teeth using the commercial whitening strips while they are wearing their retainer. Typically, if you want to use whitening strips that you purchase from the store, as opposed to professional tooth whitening products from the dentist, I would suggest you put the strips in when the retainer is not in. That way there are no issues that can arise. The strips are usually only worn for a short period of time, so you should be able to time it to where they are not on at the same time.

- **Lost Retainer.** Many people lose their retainers because they take them out, set them down and don't pay much attention to where they put them. My advice is to make sure you get in the habit of always putting your retainer in its proper case and keeping the case in a safe place. If you make it a priority to keep track of it, you shouldn't have problems with losing your retainer. But if you fail to pay attention to what you do with it, you may end up needing to purchase another one.

- **Eating.** Never wear your retainer while eating. Most Invisalign patients only wear them to bed following their treatment, but just in case you wake up in the morning and head straight to the kitchen, keep this in mind. Retainers need to be removed when eating anything. Basically, anytime your retainer is not in your mouth, it should be safe and secure in your retainer case.

- **Breakable.** It's important to handle retainers with care because they are indeed breakable. If you do break one, call your orthodontist so that you can get a replacement right away.

- **Heat.** It's not a good idea to leave your retainer in the heat, as it can damage it. If you live in a warm climate or it is summer time where you live, be sure to keep your retainer in the house, as opposed to in the car or somewhere else that it may be subjected to the warm temperatures. That way you will not run the risk of damaging your retainer from the heat.

- **Cleaning.** Your retainer should come with instructions on how to properly clean it. Typically, retainers are cleaned using toothpaste only. All you need to do is brush it clean, using your regular toothpaste. Avoid soaking your retainer in harsh cleaners. Ideally your retainer should be cleaned daily if you are wearing it each night.

- **Appointments.** Every time you go to the orthodontist, you should get in the habit of taking your retainer. This is true even if the appointment has nothing to do with the retainer. That way, if the subject comes up, there are questions, or the orthodontist wants to see it, you will have it readily available.

- **Taste.** Some people find that when they first start wearing their new retainer, it tastes weird. This is nothing to be concerned about and is only because it is new. Give it a few days and the strange new taste will wear off.

- **Flipping.** If you know anyone who wears a retainer, you may see them from time to time flip it with their tongue. This is not a good thing to do because it can damage your retainer and/or your teeth. So avoid flipping the retainer or habitually taking it in and out.

For the best long term results with your new smile, you will need to follow your orthodontist's recommendations on wearing the retainer. When it comes to determining the best retainer for you, work closely with your orthodontist. They will be able to answer those questions that are individual to you, as well as help ensure that the beautiful smile you have invested in will be long lasting!

"Today I got my Vivera retainers. My orthodontist has recommended that I wear them everyday for about the next four months. After that, I will go to only wearing the retainer at night. I've had no problems with Invisalign and I'm one very happy customer!"

- Kelly, Georgia

CHAPTER NINE:

Some advice on wisdom teeth: keeping it straight

If you have ever dealt with wisdom teeth, then this chapter may come as no surprise, yet you may still learn a little more about those molars that everyone seems to love to hate. If you, or your teen, have not yet crossed the wisdom teeth bridge, then this chapter is going to come in handy in knowing what to expect.

The History of Wisdom Teeth

Most people skate along just fine in life without any trouble from their third molars, or wisdom teeth, until one day in their late teen years or early adulthood, when it becomes an issue. It may come out of what seems like nowhere, leaving you to wonder exactly where those teeth came from!

It's a good question, too. While it seems like the wisdom teeth come from out of nowhere and just start posing a problem one day, they actually have a long established history and began making their way long before you ever noticed them. Scientists believe that the wisdom teeth once served an important purpose thousands of years ago.

Our ancestors ate a lot of food that was tougher and chewier, such as leaves, roots, and even some raw meat. It's believed that this diet was harsher on the teeth, causing them to wear down faster., Because of this, we had a third set of molars, known as the wisdom teeth today, that would erupt to help carry the burden of all that chewing.

As things changed over time, including much of our diet and the shape of our jaw, our wisdom teeth have come to pose more of a problem for most people, rather than be an asset due to the fact that they now have a difficult time fitting into our jaw. Yet not everyone even has wisdom teeth that emerge. Around 35 percent of the population never have wisdom teeth that develop, something that makes a lot of other people envious of them!

The third molars are the only teeth to completely develop after birth. There are several reasons that researchers cite for wisdom teeth that do not ever become present, which include the possibility of genetics playing a role, although that is still being researched, environmental influences, as well as trauma to the head or diseases.

What You Need to Know About Wisdom Teeth

At any given time, ask half a dozen adults around you about their wisdom teeth, and there is a good chance you will find that most have had them removed. This is common, considering what they are and some of the risks that they may pose. Many people have them removed during their younger years for valid reasons, making it a good idea to be familiar with the ins and outs of these teeth, so you will be able to deal better with them for you and your family.

What They Are, Why Removed

Wisdom teeth, also referred to as your third molars, are the larger teeth at the very back of the mouth. They are the last teeth to come in, usually somewhere between the ages of 15 and 25, which is considered to be the "age of wisdom," hence their name. While some people have no problems with their wisdom teeth erupting, many others find that they present a challenge and can be risky to the health of your other teeth.

About the time that this third set of molars begins erupting, some common problems also emerge as a result. Some of the problems associated with erupting wisdom teeth include:

- **Impaction.** According to the National Institutes of Health, wisdom teeth are the most common teeth to become impacted. When a tooth is impacted, it means that the tooth has failed to emerge through the surface of the gum or that only a portion of it has emerged.

- **Caries.** An impacted third molar leads to a high probability of creating dental caries, or cavities, both in that tooth and in the one next to it, as well. This is because they often trap plaque in the area, which is difficult to reach and to clean.

- **Cysts.** When wisdom teeth are impacted, it can cause cysts and tumors to form around the area. This can lead to additional problems because it can affect the bone, and even damage the jaw. Risks with this involve infections, as well as tooth abscesses.

- **Misalignment.** The emerging wisdom teeth may not be coming in straight or, even if they do, they can cause problems with the other teeth. As they emerge, they often push the other teeth out of alignment.

- **Discomfort.** The vast majority of people who have dealt with emerging or impacted wisdom teeth know just how uncomfortable the experience can be. From headaches to toothaches, pain, swelling, and feeling ill, the discomfort associated with wisdom teeth can make you miserable.

When to Remove

The best time to have your third set of molars removed really depends on the tooth's development. A good professional rule of thumb is to have them removed when two-thirds of the root has formed.

Ideally, it is recommended that people have them removed by the time they turn 24 years old. This is because it will help to prevent all of the problems listed above and because the ability to re-grow bone in that area of the jaw is reduced as time goes on. Also, the third set of molars is usually easier to remove when you are younger, and the recovery period is also shorter during that time.

The presence of your third set of molars is usually associated with an increased risk of periodontitis, which is an inflammation of the gums and bone, which can lead to tooth loss, abscesses, infections, and tooth shifting. It is important to note, as well, that an absence of symptoms does not mean that there is no problem or disease.

Additionally, research regarding people who did not have their wisdom teeth removed demonstrates that the older they got, the more common it was for them to have cavities in those teeth, as well as in the adjacent ones, due to the difficulties of keeping them properly cleaned. In fact, a 2011 study published in the *Journal of Oral and Maxillofacial Surgery* reported that, of the nearly 7,000 older adults they studied who had at least one third molar, most of those people had tooth decay or periodontal pathology involving those teeth, and that few had visible molars that were free of disease.

Additional Concerns

There is some controversy regarding whether those who wear a retainer or have had braces in the past need to continue wearing their retainer once the wisdom teeth have been removed. Because there is a risk of relapse if the retainer is not worn, it is recommended that patients continue wearing theirs, as recommended by their orthodontist. Doing so will help to eliminate the risks associated with shifting teeth.

If you are experiencing the emergence of your wisdom teeth, or someone in your family is, be sure you know the facts, risks, and options that are currently available. Having wisdom teeth removed is a common procedure today, and one that most people recover from without issue. Removing third molars can be an important step to take if you are having problems now, or as a preventative measure to avoid issues that can arise later.

Addressing the Issue

Either way, it is important to speak with your doctor to learn more about your specific third molar development, risks, and options. When you are dealing with your third molars, it may seem as if they steal the show, due to the discomfort they can cause. But it doesn't have to be like that since this is an issue that can usually be addressed without difficulty.

Wisdom teeth really are an issue that is better dealt with sooner, rather than later, in order to avoid a lot of discomfort, as well as the risk of an array of complications. Besides, when you address this issue head on, rather than putting it off and prolonging the issue, you will find that you gain the wisdom, without all the worry!

Wisdom Teeth and Invisalign

Understandably, many people are curious about how wisdom teeth and Invisalign fair. Some people who seek Invisalign have not yet had their third molars erupt, while others have had them extracted already, and still others may have wisdom teeth that are partially erupted.

The good news is that no matter what stage your wisdom teeth growth is in, you can still begin the Invisalign treatment program. If you have been working with your dentist about your wisdom teeth, continue to do so in order to address the issue. If the issue of your wisdom teeth arises with the orthodontist, then he or she will explain the best course of action for you to take.

It is also usually acceptable to get wisdom teeth extracted during the Invisalign treatment process. This, of course, is up to the discretion of the orthodontist you are working with, but in most cases it is acceptable. Your Invisalign aligners will be fabricated to account for wisdom teeth that are erupting and getting them extracted during the treatment process should not impede the outcome of the treatment at all.

Leaving No Stone Unturned

Now you are quite well versed on the ins and outs of both using a retainer to follow up your Invisalign treatment and wisdom teeth. It's just one more step in helping you to become comfortable and aware of the entire process. The more you know, the better prepared you will be, and that's always a good thing!

Refinements Following Treatment

Once you have completed the Invisalign treatment plan that was created for you, there is a good chance you will have to engage in what is referred to as "refinements." During the refinement phase of the treatment, any issues outside what was originally accounted for and in the treatment plan will be addressed.

For some people, this may mean wearing a few extra sets of aligners, while for others it could mean going through another dozen sets of aligners. This really varies depending on the person, their progress, and their individual treatment plan and outcome. Your orthodontist would make the recommendation on this and should be able to give you an idea of how long you will need to wear refinements.

Whether or not there will be an additional fee for the refinement aligners depends on several factors, including your orthodontist and the Invisalign treatment plan you had (e.g., Invisalign Express, Invisalign Teen, Invisalign Assist, or Invisalign Full).

Some of these treatment plans, as well as some orthodontists, do not charge for refinement, as they see it part of the overall treatment plan. So be sure to discuss this with your orthodontist ahead of time, so you know if there will be an additional charge if refinement is needed at the end of your initial treatment plan.

Here is the breakdown of the refinement inclusions for each type of Invisalign plan:

- **Invisalign Full** – Includes up to three refinements.

- **Invisalign Teen** – Includes up to three refinements.

- **Invisalign Express 10** – Allows for one refinement for purchase.

- **Invisalign Express 5** – Allows for one automated refinement for purchase.

Being a Patient Patient

Although you may be anxious to move on past the wearing of aligners, you don't want to skip past the refinement stage. It's understandable that you are anxious, it really is. But trust me when I, along with other orthodontists, advise you to be patient. If we believe you need to wear additional trays for a refinement stage, it is to help you have a more successful treatment outcome.

Believe me; you have already done the bulk of the treatment, so most of the work is done. You will be glad you finished the refinement process so that you have an even better outcome. Ask anyone who has been through it, and they will assure you that it is well worth the wait!

Advancing the Field

As you have read throughout the pages of this book, Align Technology has taken the concept of tooth alignment and has made vast improvements. They have without a doubt revolutionized the industry. But they are not done either, not by a long shot!

The company behind Invisalign, Align Technology, is continuously researching new ways to make improvements. In doing so, they have created such programs as Invisalign G3, which provides orthodontists with greater precision, more predictability on tooth movement, and efficient ClinCheck software, which allows us to reduce the number of treatment plan revisions that are needed.

As an orthodontist, we can stay on the cusp of all the new advances in the field so that we can provide our patients with the most precise treatment options. Align Technology has also introduced us to Invisalign G4, which has been designed to give us what we need to provide advanced clinical results. Invisalign G4, for example, allows for greater root tip control, improved predictability, and helps us provide an overall superior clinical outcome.

This is great news for the consumer. When you work with your orthodontist, you can take comfort in knowing that he or she is working with the most advanced system that there is for aligning teeth. They are also working with the most precise system, which has a high success rate. Invisalign is an advanced system that is accurate, uniquely tailored, and quite simply, hard to beat.

Choosing Invisalign, any of their programs, means that you are choosing to put your trust in a treatment system that has proven, with well over 1.5 million people so far, that it is well deserving of all the attention and popularity it is receiving. It has earned its reputation by providing a high-quality, accurate, and dependable treatment that helps people achieve the beautiful smile they want!

CHAPTER TEN:
Celebrate Your New Smile

Throughout the pages of this book, we have focused a lot on how working with an orthodontist your teeth can become straight. We have even discussed the importance of having straight teeth as it relates to some health issues. But we have only briefly touched on the social aspect of having a great smile, or at least one that you feel good about showing.

In this final chapter, we are going to look at the social implications of having a smile that make someone feel confident, as well as what some of the issues are that are associated with people not feeling confident about their smile.

We will conclude this chapter with a look at ways that you can celebrate your new smile once you finish your Invisalign treatment. As you have learned throughout this book, and as you will continue to find, having a great smile can do a lot for you in terms of helping you feel confident and comfortable.

The Great Smile

Many people believe that the smile is a universal language. It's something that we all do, no matter where in the world we are from, even if it may have slightly different meanings that are dictated by culture. Still, it's something that we all do throughout the world.

In America, a smile is seen as a gesture of kindness and friendliness. Just consider for a moment how a smile impacts your life. Giving someone a smile can make the difference in one's day, or turning a situation around to make it more pleasant. There is a lot of power in such a simple thing as the smile!

But what happens if that smile is riddled with teeth that look unsightly? What if when the person smiles you are able to see teeth that are misaligned or even rotted or severely out of place? Often times what happens to the observer is that they don't see the friendly smile that was intended. Instead, they notice the teeth and concentrate on them. That's not the intention most people have when they give a smile.

What's more, over time, those who have a smile that they don't feel great about may lose self confidence. They may withdraw or shy away from social opportunities. They may not want to talk as much, so they don't have to worry about people seeing their teeth. You may have even seen people who will laugh in a conversation, and they put their hand up to cover their mouth, embarrassed about their teeth or smile.

Seeking Change

Simply by reading this book it shows you are interested in leaving behind all that comes with a smile you are not completely comfortable with. Truth be told, straightening your teeth and working to get a smile you feel great about is not something you are ever likely to look back upon and regret. It would be rare to find people who have corrected their teeth and regret having done so.

However, it is not difficult to find people who regret never taking the first step toward a spectacular smile. Some people put it off, pass it up, and assume they are too old, too broke, or whatever other excuses enter their mind. But they still go on to regret not having taken the steps necessary to fix their teeth. As a result of this, they have in some cases sold themselves short and may have a lot of missed opportunity. Many people who have crooked or crowded teeth tend to refrain from social activities, miss out on job promotions and are judged to be less friendly, to be less educated and to have a low socio-economic situation. It isn't fair, but the point remains that your smile says a lot about you.

Social Implications

While you and I have an idea that there are social downfalls to not having nice straight teeth, many people may not even realize that their teeth are the reason they are struggling in other areas of their life. Believe it or not, the teeth have a powerful connection to so many aspects of our life and what we will go on to do and not do.

Oral health is something that we all need to be concerned with because it has such health and social implications. Oral health can include tooth decay, gum disease, and even facial pain that some people may experience from having issues with their teeth.

When it comes to oral health:

- An October 2010 study in the *American Journal of Public Health* found that children who have poor oral health were more likely to miss school and perform poorly in school.

- Researchers at DePauw University reported on a correlation between one's smile in pictures and how happy they would be later in life. They found that even by looking at the photographs of children at the age of five they could often predict accurately if the person would go on to later be divorced in life. Those that didn't smile in family pictures growing up tended to have more divorces and live unhappier lives as an adult.

- A July 2011 article in the *Los Angeles Times* shared information research conducted regarding the social implications of the smile, as well as straight teeth. What the researchers found is that people feel more negatively toward those with rotted teeth, as well as crooked teeth. Using the same photos of a group of teens, one version showing them with straight teeth and one without, study participants rated those with straight teeth 10 percent higher across the board. The conclusion of the research indicated that there is a social benefit to having straight teeth.

- In the field of social psychology, it is held that nice teeth, which include them being white and straight, are considered to be a sign of attractiveness.

- A survey conducted by the American Academy of Cosmetic Dentistry found that around 92 percent of adults polled felt that having an attractive smile was socially important. Nearly as many people felt that an unattractive smile made the person less appealing. What's more, they found that around 75 percent of the people believed that an unattractive smile was detrimental to one's career success.

- The same poll that was conducted above also found that half of the people who participated believed that unattractive teeth were a sign of poor personal hygiene.

- Overall, the belief is that those who have an unattractive smile, for whatever reason, are going to be more likely to experience discrimination when it comes to employment, as well as in social situations.

As you can see, our teeth play a big role in our social life. It even makes a difference when it comes to our rating of a stranger's likeability. If they have nice teeth and a pleasant smile, we are more likely to find them friendlier and more likeable. Sure, this may not be fair. I realize you may be thinking this. But this is not something that is necessarily planned out or taught. It's just the way our culture, along with many others, happen to be.

The truth of the matter is that teeth are a big part of our social life. Having a great smile is associated with high social status, which will often help people do better on a job interview, be more comfortable on a first date, and even do better in school or work around their peers and colleagues.

Benefits Galore

There are so many positive social benefits of having a great smile. There is a good chance that even before reading this book you had an idea that this was true. You may even be able to point to several places in your own life where not having straight teeth has negatively impacted you. If you can... great!

Because you can rest assure knowing that once you go through the Invsalign treatment, you will never feel that way again.

Some of the social benefits of having a great smile include:

- A nice smile makes us more attractive. This is true when people look at us, but it also makes us feel more attractive to begin with.

- When we have a smile we are proud of, we are more likely to show it. Smiling lifts our mood and makes us happy. Even if you are feeling down, if you sit and smile for a couple of minutes, it will send cues to your body that you are happy, and you will begin feeling happy.

- When we smile more, we also relieve stress, and who couldn't use some stress relief?

- Having a great smile will make you feel more confident. This confidence can transcend throughout many areas of your life, including jobs, school, and personal relationships. Being more confident in these areas can help lead you to more success.

- People often judge people by their smile, and if you have a great one, they are likely to find you more attractive, trusting, successful, honest, likeable, and more successful.

- Those who are considered to be attractive end up making more money, up to 27 percent more, than those people considered unattractive.

Fixing your teeth, as I often tell my patients, is well worth the return on investment. It is difficult for people to grasp that idea right off. But when you look at the benefits that arise from straightening your teeth, it is clear to see that the return on investment really is amazing. Just think – what else can you invest around $5,000 into and come out with opportunities for better jobs, more meaningful social relationships, being more attractive, and feeling more confident as you go through the rest of your life? You are right, not much! Straightening your teeth is well worth the benefits that you get in return.

Next, assuming you are going to go through with straightening your teeth, I'd like to give you an idea about how you, or your teen, can celebrate after finishing the Invisalign treatment.

7 Ways to Celebrate Finishing Your Invisalign Treatment

Having Invisalign, or braces, on your teeth can be a treatment that can last for a year or more, depending upon all the factors. And during the time that you have had them on your teeth, you might have felt like you missed out on a lot!

There are things you couldn't eat at all following an adjustment or new set of trays, due to sore teeth.

Time to Celebrate

So the day is finally in sight. It's time to get the Invisalign, or braces, off and celebrate your new smile. Now is the time to celebrate! There are so many ways that you can celebrate, everything from writing a journal about your experience to recording a video that shares your experience and shows your new look.

Here are seven options that you may want to consider:

1. **Throw a party.** Throwing a treatment is over party is a great way to celebrate. Invite your friends over and enjoy showing off those new straight teeth. Your friends will love being able to take part in your celebration.

2. **Plan a photo shoot.** You deserve to show the world your new beautiful smile! Plan a photo shoot, so you can be one-on-one with a photographer and put your best smile forward. You will get some great shots and can show all your MySpace of Facebook friends your new look. You may even want to complete the whole look by making your photo shoot one of the glamour shot ones, where

you get the make-up and hair pampering right before the shoot.

3. **Chew some gum.** You know you have been wanting to chew gum for the longest time. Although it's not a good thing to still do regularly, you can take an afternoon and have some gum and feel guilt and worry free. Chew to your heart's content!

4. **Go caramel.** Now is the time that you can sink your teeth into a caramel apple. No more avoiding the caramel and cutting the apple into bite-sized pieces or having to remove your aligner. Nope, you can actually eat a full caramel apple, right off the stick! Get one at the mall, a carnival, or have fun making them yourself. Either way, you will love being able to bite into that sticky, gooey sweetness worry free!

5. **Picnic in the park.** Weather permitting, a picnic in the park will make for a fun celebration. Take some of your favorite outdoor games, invite the friends, and have a cooler filled with icy drinks. On the grill, you can plan for things like corn on the cob that you were probably avoiding throughout treatment. It will make for a memorable afternoon!

6. **Throw a potluck party.** Have your friends each bring a dish people with braces have to take precaution with.

This will give them the chance to learn a little more about what you went through, and it will be fun to see what options they come up with. Ask each of your guests to write down one comment about you with or without your braces. Your potluck will be filled with interesting dishes, laughs, and a good time!

7. **Hit the spa.** What could be better then spending a couple of hours being pampered? Not much! Have a spa party for yourself, or invite a friend or two. Get a makeover, manicure, pedicure, massage, or whatever else you feel like getting. Just pamper yourself for making it through your treatment. You will walk out feeling and looking great!

Doing some of the above things, such as chewing gum, may still not be good for your teeth or your body overall. But doing it on a special occasion, and not making a habit out of it, shouldn't do any harm.

Looking Ahead

Now that you have made it through wearing your Invisalign aligners, you will find that you like to smile more, show off your beautiful teeth, and feel great! Having a celebration for getting your braces off is a great way to remember the day as something really special, include those you love, and start a new you!

There are many ways to celebrate. Think outside the box and determine what way will work best for you. Perhaps you want to have friends over, make it a family affair, or you just want to celebrate alone. Whichever way you choose to do it, it will be a special day!

Final Thoughts

As an orthodontist, I see people on a daily basis that wish to change their smile. They walk into my office knowing that they need to do something, but may not know where to begin. For the many people who I have provided Invisalign treatment to, I have witnessed their transformation.

People may begin wondering if Invisalign is the right choice for them, but once they get it, and especially after they have completed it, they know the answer without a doubt. It's a resounding yes. Invisalign offers people an advanced method of tooth alignment that will help give you the smile you want. It's affordable, precise, effective, and is a great treatment for those who are serious about creating an amazing smile.

With Invisalign, you leave behind the negatives associated with braces, and you gain the positives that the system, and tooth alignment, provides. You simply can't go wrong with

Invisalign. I wish you the best of luck with your own Invisalign journey!

GLOSSARY

3D layering – Another term for stereolithography, which is the process that Invisalign uses to create the aligners that are worn during treatment. It's a process that allows for making a solid object out of a computer image.

Align Technology – The company that makes theInvisalign System. The company was startedin 1997 by Zia Chishti and Kelsey Wirth, inPalo Alto, California. Today they areheadquartered in Santa Clara, California, andhave over 800 employees that workthroughout the U.S., Costa Rica, Mexico, and Europe.

Aligners - Clear plastic custom-fitted trays that are used during the Invisalign treatment process in order to align teeth. Patients first undergo a process that allows for gathering information about the person's current tooth alignment, as well as where it should be. The information is then used to create a series of aligners that the patient will wear to correct the tooth alignment.

AutoBite – A tool used during the making of the Invisalign aligners that was created in 2003. This tool increased the bite accuracy to 99 percent.

Bite registration – A process of getting an impression of the person's bite. It's done by using a dental caulk that the patient will bite down on.

Bleaching teeth – The process of making teeth whiter and brighter. This process can often be completed in conjunction with Invisalign treatment.

Blue dot – A dot system that is used on the Invisalign Teen aligners, so that you can easily verify if it is time to move on to the next set of aligners.

BPA -Stands for bisphenol A, which is an industrial chemical, often found in plastics. The Invisalign aligners are BPA free, so they do not contain the substance.

Bruxism -The process of clenching and grinding the teeth. It can cause problems, such as temporomandibular joint disorder (TMJ-D). Retainers are sometimes used to help address the condition.

Caries -Tooth decay or a cavity, considered to be one of the most common conditions in the world. They are usually treated with fillings or crowns.

Computerized tomography – The process of taking an image of the teeth. It uses advanced 3D imaging to make the pictures.

ClinCheck - Software used by the doctor to see a 3D representation of the treatment plan that the patient will be following. The software allows the doctor to review the plan and make changes as needed.

Cysts - When wisdom teeth are impacted, it can cause cysts and tumors to form around the area. This can lead to additional problems because it can affect the bone, and even damage the jaw. Risks with this involve infections, as well as tooth abscesses.

Dental appliance – Those items that are used to correct an issue with the mouth or teeth, including Invisalign, braces, retainers, etc.

Eruption tabs - The Invisalign teen aligners have been designed to have "eruption tabs" to account for the patient's erupting second molars.

Flexible spending account - Many employers have FSAs options, where a designated portion of your paycheck would go into the account. The funds are there to pay for qualified medical expenses, which may include Invisalign treatment.

Flipping - The process of flipping the retainer that people wear. Some people like to flip the retainer in and out of their mouth, but it can damage both the teeth and the retainer.

Fixed retainer - A fixed retainer is typically bonded to the inside surfaces of the lower front teeth. This type of retainer can be attached to the two canine teeth or to every tooth in the area.

Gingivitis – Gingivitis is an inflammation of the gums that can result from poor dental hygiene. It can also result from misaligned teeth. If your teeth are crowded or not aligned properly, you may have a difficult time being able to properly clean them, especially in between them, which will allow the plaque to build up.

Hygiene aides – Each Invisalign Starter Kit comes with hygiene aides, which will help keep teeth and aligners clean.

Impaction - Wisdom teeth are the most common teeth to become impacted. When a tooth is impacted, it means that the tooth has failed to emerge through the surface of the gum or that only a portion of it has emerged.

Interproximal reduction - This is a process that is used to reduce the size of the enamel between the teeth. It is often performed when teeth are crowded.

Invisalign - The tooth alignment treatment system that over 1.5 million people have opted for. It offers a nearly invisible route to tooth alignment, along with the most advanced technology available, which will help ensure accuracy and successful treatment.

Invisalign Assist - This is a product support option that is offered throughout the Invisalign treatment. It helps people be able to achieve their aesthetic goals better with their Invisalign plan. It helps with progress tracking, appointment plans, and has compliance indicators. This treatment plan takes 6 to 12 months, includes up to three refinements, but does not include any mid-course corrections.

Invisalign Express 5 - This is a program for those with minor issues, such as mild spacing, crowding, or other orthodontic issues. While using the same Invisalign technology, the treatment takes about 2.5 months, includes one automated refinement for purchase, but does not allow for mid-course correction.

Invisalign Express 10 - This is a program that works just like the full program, only is a shorter one. It's typically for people who need only minor alignment corrections. The treatment can usually be completed within six months. It allows for purchasing one refinement but does not allow for mid-course correction.

Invisalign Full - This is the full program that has been described in-depth throughout this book. It generally takes 6 to 12 months for the treatment, allows up to three refinements that are included, and allows for a mid-course correction for a fee.

Invisalign Teen - This program, as discussed, has been designed for the growing teenager. Treatment takes 12 to 18 months, three refinements are included, and mid-course correction is available for a fee. It also includes six free replacement aligners for those that are lost or damaged.

Metal braces - These are traditional braces that involve using metal wires and brackets that are affixed to the teeth and used in the alignment process.

Mid-course correction - When the original treatment plan must be re-planned in order to compensate for some changes that have taken place with your mouth or teeth. This may happen as a result of you having some dental work, such as fillings, or from some type of trauma that has occurred. If this does happen, it requires additional work in creating a new treatment plan, so there is usually a charge incurred.

Misalignment - This is the term for teeth that are not in proper alignment. They may be crooked, crowded, spaced too far, etc.

Orthodontist – A specialist in teeth straightening, who has completed 2-3 years of training beyond dental school.

Overbite - A condition where the top teeth tend to excessively overlap the lower teeth. This is a condition that orthodontists find easy to correct.

Pontic - An artificial tooth on a dental bridge. They are added to retainers in place of missing teeth.

Refinement - A phase at the end of the Invisalign treatment process. During the refinement phase of the treatment, any issues outside what was originally accounted for and in the treatment plan will be addressed.

Removeable retainer - This is a type of retainer that is removable, rather than being affixed to the teeth.

Root resorption - The process where there has been a breakdown and loss of the tooth's root structure.

Stereolithography - This is a computerized process that allows for creating a three-dimensional replica of the mouth and teeth.

Starter kit - This is the kit that is given out with the first set of aligners. It will contain hygiene items, a storage case, as well as other helpful information.

Third molars - This is another term for the wisdom teeth. Many people find that their wisdom teeth cause problems and they need to have them removed.

Underbite - A condition where the lower teeth grow and extend beyond the upper teeth. This occurs less frequently than an overbite. Medically it is also referred to as mandilbula prognathia.

Veneers - A layer that goes over the teeth in an effort to restore it and make it look more aesthetically appealing.

Vivera retainers - The line of retainers that have been created by Align Technology, the same company that created Invisalign.

Wisdom teeth - The third set of molars that often grow in the far back of the mouth.

INDEX

CPSIA information can be obtained at www.ICGtesting.com
Printed in the USA
BVOW07*0908260814

364295BV00012B/561/P